WHO Global Influenza
Surveillance Network

Manual for the laboratory diagnosis and virological surveillance of influenza

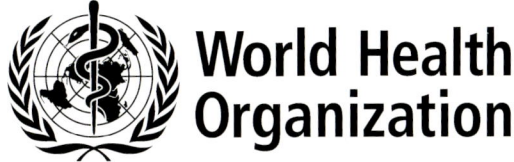

WHO Library Cataloguing-in-Publication Data

Manual for the laboratory diagnosis and virological surveillance of influenza.

1.Influenza, Human – epidemiology. 2.Influenza, Human – virology. 3.Influenza, Human – diagnosis. 4.Immunologic Tests – methods. 5.Population surveillance – methods. 6.Pandemics – prevention and control. 7.Serologic tests – methods. 8.Practice guideline. I.World Health Organization. II.Title:WHO global influenza surveillance network: manual for the laboratory diagnosis and virological surveillance of influenza.

ISBN 978 92 4 154809 0 (NLM classification: WC 515)

© World Health Organization 2011

All rights reserved. Publications of the World Health Organization can be obtained from WHO Press, World Health Organization, 20 Avenue Appia, 1211 Geneva 27, Switzerland (tel.: +41 22 791 3264; fax: +41 22 791 4857; e-mail: bookorders@who.int). Requests for permission to reproduce or translate WHO publications – whether for sale or for noncommercial distribution – should be addressed to WHO Press, at the above address (fax: +41 22 791 4806; e-mail: permissions@who.int).

The designations employed and the presentation of the material in this publication do not imply the expression of any opinion whatsoever on the part of the World Health Organization concerning the legal status of any country, territory, city or area or of its authorities, or concerning the delimitation of its frontiers or boundaries. Dotted lines on maps represent approximate border lines for which there may not yet be full agreement.

The mention of specific companies or of certain manufacturers' products does not imply that they are endorsed or recommended by the World Health Organization in preference to others of a similar nature that are not mentioned. Errors and omissions excepted, the names of proprietary products are distinguished by initial capital letters.

All reasonable precautions have been taken by the World Health Organization to verify the information contained in this publication. However, the published material is being distributed without warranty of any kind, either expressed or implied. The responsibility for the interpretation and use of the material lies with the reader. In no event shall the World Health Organization be liable for damages arising from its use.

Designed by minimum graphics
Printed in Malta

Contents

Acknowledgements	v
Glossary	vi
List of contacts	vii
Objectives of the WHO manual	ix
Abbreviations	xi

Part 1: The virology and epidemiology, control and surveillance of influenza — 1

1.A	Influenza virology and epidemiology	3
1.B	Influenza control	11
1.C	Influenza surveillance	15

Part 2: The laboratory diagnosis and virological surveillance of influenza — 27

2.A	Collection, storage and transport of specimens	29
2.B	Processing of clinical specimens for virus isolation	33
2.C	Virus isolation in cell culture	35
2.D	Virus isolation and passage in embryonated chicken eggs	39
2.E	Identification of the haemagglutinin subtype of viral isolates by haemagglutination inhibition testing	43
2.F	Serological diagnosis of influenza by haemagglutination inhibition testing	59
2.G	Serological diagnosis of influenza by microneutralization assay	63
2.H	Identification of neuraminidase subtype by neuraminidase assay and neuraminidase inhibition test	79
2.I	Molecular identification of influenza isolates	83
2.J	Virus identification by immunofluorescence antibody staining	97
2.K	Use of neuraminidase inhibition assays to determine the susceptibility of influenza viruses to antiviral drugs	103

References — 115

Bibliography		**117**
	Influenza surveillance	117
	Influenza control	118
	Biosaftey	119
	Collection and transport of clinical specimens	119
	Detection of influenza virus and antibodies	119
	A(H5) outbreaks	121
	Haemagglutination and haemagglutination inhibition	121
	Molecular analysis	121

Annexes		**123**
Annex I	Laboratory safety	125
Annex II	Cell culture inoculation and passage worksheet	127
Annex III	Egg inoculation record	128
Annex IV	Influenza antigen standardization worksheet	129
Annex V	Haemagglutination inhibition test results – field isolate identification	130
Annex VI	Haemagglutination inhibition test results – serological diagnosis	132
Annex VII	Microneutralization assay process sheet	133
Annex VIII	Calculation of neuraminidase inhibition titre (NAI_{50})	137

Acknowledgements

This manual was jointly developed by five World Health Organization Collaborating Centres (WHOCCs) for influenza (the WHOCC for Reference and Research on Influenza, Melbourne, Australia; the WHOCC for Reference and Research on Influenza, Tokyo, Japan; the WHOCC for Reference and Research on Influenza, London, United Kingdom; the WHOCC for Surveillance, Epidemiology and Control of Influenza, Atlanta, United States; and the WHOCC for Studies on the Ecology of Influenza in Animals, Memphis, United States.

The special contribution of the WHOCC for Surveillance, Epidemiology and Control of Influenza in Atlanta is acknowledged, in particular the efforts of Henrietta Hall and Thomas Rowe in preparing the manual, and of Nancy Cox and Alexandra Klimov in its primary reviewing and editing.

WHO also wishes to acknowledge the contributions of three national reference laboratories (the Therapeutic Goods Administration Laboratories, Canberra, Australia; the National Institute for Biological Standards and Control, London, United Kingdom; and the Centre for Biologics Evaluation and Research, Rockville, United States) and of the National Influenza Centre, China, Hong Kong Special Administrative Region. The sharing by influenza experts of laboratory protocols for the diagnosis of pandemic (H1N1) 2009 in humans is also acknowledged.

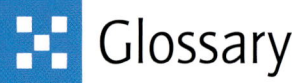 Glossary

Antigenic drift – the gradual alteration by point mutations of the haemagglutinin (HA) and neuraminidase (NA) proteins within a type or subtype which results in the inability of antibodies to previous strains to neutralize the mutant virus. Antigenic drift occurs in both influenza A and B viruses and causes periodic epidemics.

Antigenic shift – the appearance in the human population of an influenza A virus containing a novel HA protein with or without a novel NA protein that are immunologically different from those of isolates circulating previously. Antigenic shift is responsible for worldwide pandemics.

Disease surveillance – the systematic, continuing assessment of the health of a community, based on the collection, interpretation and use of health data. Surveillance provides information necessary for public health decision-making.

Epidemiology – the study of the distribution and determinants of health-related states or events in specified populations, and the application of this study to the control of health problems.

Influenza epidemic – an outbreak of influenza caused by influenza A or B viruses that have undergone antigenic drift. The terms "influenza epidemic" and "influenza outbreak" have the same meaning, and may occur locally or in many parts of the world during the same season.

Influenza pandemic – by convention, worldwide outbreaks of influenza caused by influenza A viruses that have undergone antigenic shift. However, as recently demonstrated, an antigenically novel virus of an existing subtype is capable of pandemic spread

Virological surveillance – the ongoing and systematic collection and analysis of viruses in order to monitor their characteristics.

List of contacts

World Health Organization

Global Influenza Programme (GIP)
Health Security and Environment (HSE)
Avenue Appia 20, 1211 Geneva 27, Switzerland

Dr Wenqing Zhang, Team Leader: Virus Monitoring, Assessment and Vaccine Support Unit, GIP/HSE
Dr Terry G. Besselaar: Virus Monitoring, Assessment and Vaccine Support Unit, GIP/HSE

E-mail: gisn@who.int
Fax: +41 22 791 4878
www.who.int/influenza

WHO Collaborating Centres for Influenza

Australia

WHO Collaborating Centre for Reference and Research on Influenza
10 Wreckyn Street, North Melbourne, Victoria 3051, Australia

Dr Anne Kelso, Director
Dr Ian Barr (contact)

E-mail: Ian.Barr@influenzacentre.org
Fax: +61 3 9342 3939
www.influenzacentre.org

China

WHO Collaborating Centre for Reference and Research on Influenza
National Institute for Viral Disease control and Prevention, Chinese Center for Disease Control and Prevention, 155 Changbai Road, Changping District, 102206, Beijing, China

Dr Yuelong Shu, Director
Dr Dayan Wang (contact)

E-mail: yshu@cnic.org.cn
Fax: +86 10 5890 0851
http://www.cnic.org.cn

Japan

WHO Collaborating Centre for Reference and Research on Influenza
National Institute of Infectious Diseases
Department of Virology III
4-7-1 Gakuen, Musashi-Murayama-shi, Tokyo 208-0011, Japan

Dr Masato Tashiro, Director
Dr Takato Odagiri (contact)

E-mail: todagiri@nih.go.jp
Fax: +81 42 561 0812
http://idsc.nih.go.jp/index.html

United Kingdom

WHO Collaborating Centre for Reference and Research on Influenza
National Institute for Medical Research
Mill Hill, London NW7 1AA, United Kingdom

Dr John McCauley, Director
Dr Rod Daniels (contact)

E-mail: whocc@nimr.mrc.ac.uk
Fax: +44 208 906 4477
www.nimr.mrc.ac.uk/wic/

United States

WHO Collaborating Centre for Surveillance, Epidemiology and Control of Influenza
Centers for Disease Control and Prevention
Influenza Branch
1600 Clifton Road, G16, Atlanta, GA 30333, USA

Dr Nancy Cox, Director
Dr Alexander Klimov (contact)

E-mail: axk0@cdc.gov
Fax: +1 404 639 0080; +1 404 639 3378
www.cdc.gov/flu/

United States

WHO Collaborating Centre for Studies on The Ecology of Influenza in Animals
St. Jude Children's Research Hospital
262 Danny Thomas Place, Memphis TN 38105-2794, USA

Dr Richard Webby (contact)

E-mail: richard.webby@stjude.org
Fax: +1 901 595 8559
www.stjude.org

Objectives of the WHO manual

In many settings influenza is recognized as a major cause of disease and death. In other parts of the world, however, its epidemiology and the degree of its impact on human health remain relatively uncertain – in large part due to a lack of virological and disease surveillance.

WHO continues to work to increase awareness of the importance of influenza as a cause of disease and death worldwide, and to increase understanding of the importance, organization and goals of the WHO Global Influenza Surveillance Network (GISN). Surveillance is the foundation underpinning all efforts to understand, prevent and control influenza, and global influenza surveillance – initiated in 1952 – has long provided the information needed each year to select the precise virus strains to be used as the basis of annual vaccines. Such surveillance activities also provide the vital information needed to establish the degree of seasonality of influenza in various parts of the world, and to estimate its impact and burden.

In addition, global influenza surveillance forms the primary line of defence against the occurrence of influenza pandemics by identifying emerging influenza virus strains that pose a potential threat. The importance of this has been demonstrated on numerous occasions, for example in 1997, 2003 and 2004 when influenza A(H5N1) viruses were detected in humans in China, Hong Kong Special Administrative Region (Hong Kong SAR); in 1999 when A(H9N2) was identified in Hong Kong SAR; in 2003 when A(H7N7) was detected in the Netherlands; in 2004 when A(H5N1) was detected in south-east Asia (with subsequent spread to other regions); and in 2009 with the emergence of the declared pandemic of A(H1N1) influenza.

An integral part of GISN activities is the laboratory diagnosis and virological surveillance of circulating influenza viruses – key elements in both influenza vaccine virus selection and the early detection of emerging viruses with pandemic potential.

WHO has therefore developed this manual in order to strengthen the laboratory diagnosis and virological surveillance of influenza infection by providing standard methods for the collection, detection, isolation and characterization of viruses. The specific objectives of the manual include:

- increasing understanding of the principles and importance of haemagglutination and haemagglutination inhibition (HAI) testing in the identification of influenza virus field isolates, and in serological diagnosis using the WHO Influenza Reagent Kit;
- ensuring HAI test results are analysed and interpreted accurately by including the appropriate controls and recognizing potential problems in interpreting test results;

- increasing understanding of the principles of reverse transcription polymerase chain reaction (RT-PCR) and its application in the typing and subtyping of influenza viruses;
- highlighting the significance of influenza virus isolation as compared with direct antigen detection;
- increasing understanding of the principles of the microneutralization assay and its application to serological diagnosis;
- increasing understanding of the principles of the neuraminidase inhibition (NAI) assays used in the detection of virus strains resistant to antivirals.

All national and international influenza surveillance systems – including those for monitoring clinical disease – depend fundamentally upon the consistent and successful implementation of the key laboratory activities in these and other areas described in this manual.

Disclaimer

Throughout this manual, the mention of specific companies or of certain manufacturers' products does not imply that they are endorsed or recommended by the World Health Organization in preference to others of a similar nature that are not mentioned. Similar products from other companies that are available locally can instead be used.

Abbreviations

2-TBA	2-thiobarbituric acid
cat. no.	catalogue number
CCs	cell controls
cDNA	complementary DNA
CPE	cytopathic effect
D-MEM	Dulbecco's Modified Eagle Medium
DNA	deoxyribonucleic acid
DNTP	deoxyribonucleoside triphosphate
EDTA	ethylene diamine tetraacetic acid
ELISA	enzyme-linked immunosorbent assay
FBS	fetal bovine serum
FG	French gauge
FITC	fluorescein isothiocyanate
HA	haemagglutinin
HA_d	haemadsorption
HAI	haemagglutination inhibition
HEPES	*N*-2-hydroxyethylpiperazine-*N*'-2-ethane sulfonic acid
HRP	horseradish peroxidase
IC_{50}	drug concentration needed to inhibit neuraminidase activity by 50%
IFA	immunofluorescence antibody
ILI	influenza-like illness
M gene	gene coding for matrix protein (M1) and transmembrane protein (M2)
MDCK	Madin-Darby canine kidney
NA	neuraminidase
NAI	neuraminidase inhibition
NP	nucleoprotein
NS gene	gene coding for non-structural protein
NTC	negative template control
OD	optical density
OPD	o-phenylenediamine dihydrochloride
PBS	phosphate-buffered saline
PCR	polymerase chain reaction
PTC	positive template control
RBC	red blood cell
RDE	receptor destroying enzyme

RFLP	restriction fragment length polymorphism
RNA	ribonucleic acid
RNP	RNase P
RT	reverse transcription
RT-PCR	reverse transcription polymerase chain reaction
TBE	Tris-Borate-EDTA buffer
$TCID_{50}$	50% tissue culture infectious dose
TPCK	tosylphenylalanylchloromethane
VCs	virus controls

PART 1
The virology and epidemiology, control and surveillance of influenza

1.A
Influenza virology and epidemiology

Influenza viruses

Influenza viruses (**FIGURE 1.A-1**) belong to the *Orthomyxoviridae* family and are divided into types A, B and C. Influenza types A and B are responsible for epidemics of respiratory illness that are often associated with increased rates of hospitalization and death. Influenza type C is not discussed in this manual as it is a milder infection that does not cause epidemics, and does not therefore have the severe public health impact of influenza types A and B.

All influenza viruses are negative-strand RNA viruses with a segmented genome. As shown in **FIGURE 1.A-2** Influenza type A and B viruses have 8 genes that code for 10 proteins, including the surface proteins haemagglutinin (HA) and neuraminidase (NA). In the case of influenza type A viruses, further subdivision can be made into different subtypes according to differences in these two surface proteins. To date, 16 HA subtypes and 9 NA subtypes have been identified. However, during the 20th century, the only influenza A subtypes that circulated extensively in humans were A(H1N1); A(H1N2); A(H2N2); and A(H3N2). All known subtypes of influenza type A viruses have been isolated from birds and can affect a range of mammal species. As with humans, the number of influenza A subtypes that have been isolated from other mammalian species is limited. Influenza type B viruses almost exclusively infect humans.

The hallmark of human influenza viruses is their ability to undergo antigenic change, which occurs in the following two ways:

- ■ ***Antigenic drift*** – is a process of gradual and relatively continuous change in the viral HA and NA proteins. It results from the accumulation of point mutations in the HA and NA genes during viral replication. Both influenza type A and B viruses undergo antigenic drift, leading to new virus strains. The emergence of these new strains necessitates the frequent updating of influenza vaccine virus strains. Because antibodies to previous influenza infections may not provide full protection against the new strains resulting from antigenic drift, individuals can have many influenza infections over a lifetime.

FIGURE 1.A-1
Electron micrograph of influenza type A viruses[a]

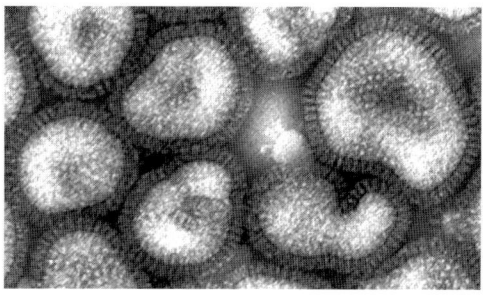

[a] Reproduced by permission of Dr K Gopal Murti and Dr R Webster, St Jude Children's Research Hospital.

FIGURE 1.A-2
Structure of the influenza virus[a]

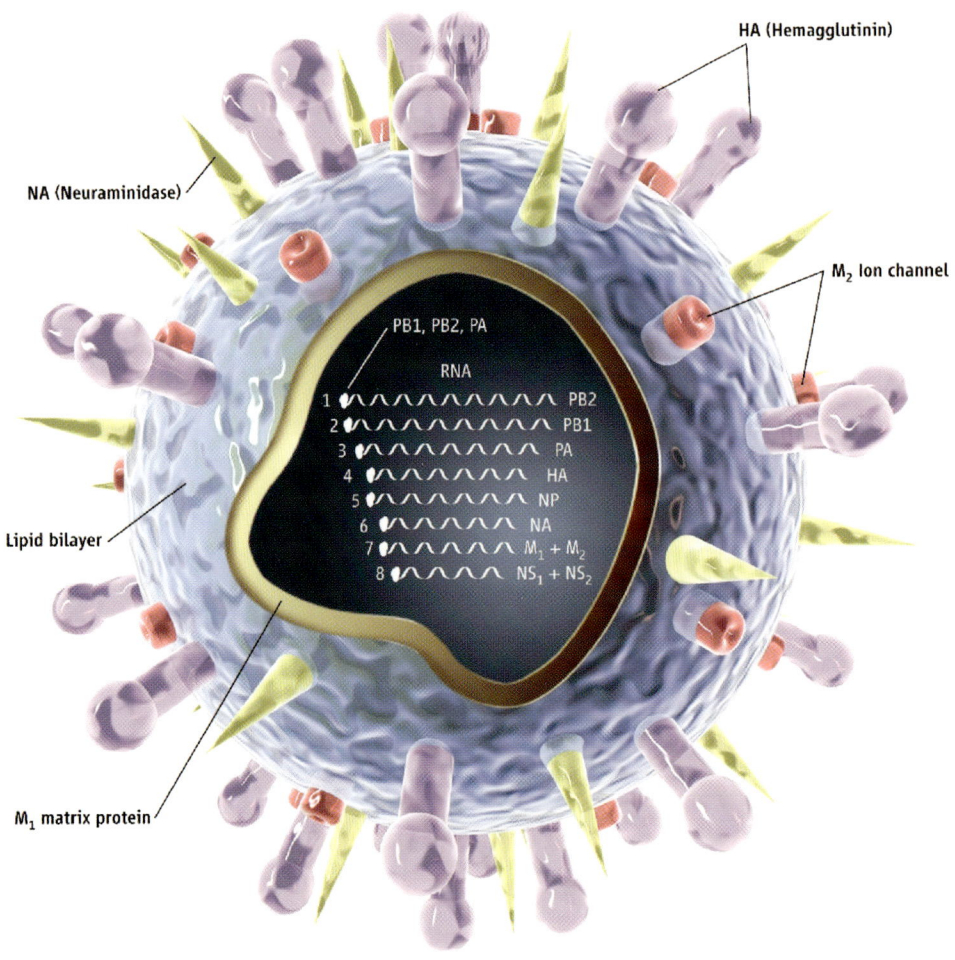

Key for the proteins encoded by the 8 influenza genes
HA   haemagglutinin protein
NA   neuraminidase protein
M_1 matrix protein
M_2 transmembrane protein
NP   nucleoprotein
NS_1 and NS_2 non-structural proteins
PA   polymerase A
PB1   polymerase B1
PB2   polymerase B2

[a] Chris Bickel/*Science*. Reprinted with permission from *Science* (21 April 2006) 312: 380. © AAAS, 2006. *Readers may view, browse, and/or download material for temporary copying purposes only, provided these uses are for noncommercial personal purposes. Except as provided by law, this material may not be further reproduced, distributed, transmitted, modified, adapted, performed, displayed, published, or sold in whole or in part, without written prior permission from the publisher.*

- ***Antigenic shift*** – in addition to antigenic drift, influenza type A viruses can also undergo a more dramatic and abrupt type of change called antigenic shift. By definition, a shift has occurred when an influenza type A virus emerges among humans bearing either a HA protein or a combination of HA and NA proteins that have not been circulating among humans in recent years. There are at least three possible mechanisms by which antigenic shift can occur:
    1. a virus bearing new HA and NA proteins can arise through the genetic reassortment of non-human and human influenza viruses;
    2. an influenza virus from other animals (e.g. birds or pigs) can infect a human directly without undergoing genetic reassortment; or
    3. a non-human virus may be passed from one type of animal (e.g. birds) through an intermediate animal host (such as a pig) to humans.

Whereas antigenic drift occurs continuously, antigenic shift occurs infrequently and unpredictably. Since antigenic shift results in the emergence of a new influenza virus, a large proportion (or even all) of the world's population will have no antibodies against it. If the new strain is capable of causing illness in humans and sustained chains of human-to-human transmission leading to community-wide outbreaks then such a virus has the potential to spread worldwide, causing a pandemic.

Spread of influenza

Influenza viruses are spread from infectious people to susceptible people through large virus-containing droplets and aerosols that are produced by coughing, sneezing or talking. Less commonly, influenza viruses may also be spread via contaminated fomites or by direct touching. Children are an important factor in the spread of influenza within communities and within households – influenza outbreaks among schoolchildren can herald the start of influenza activity in a community. During some community outbreaks, illness rates among school-age children have been shown to rise and decline earlier in the outbreak than the rates among adults. Households with young children have higher influenza illness rates overall and secondary attack rates are higher in households where the index case is a young child. In addition to exposure to influenza in households, exposure to influenza in other closed settings can also be associated with high attack rates. Reported examples include outbreaks in nursing homes and hospital wards (Arden et al., 1995), among passengers on a cruise ship (Brotherton et al., 2003) and among adolescents in a ski hostel (Lyytikäinen et al., 1998).

Epidemiology of seasonal influenza

Although epidemics of influenza occur almost every year in temperate climates, the rates and severity of illness caused can vary substantially from year to year. The severity of annual epidemics is affected by several factors including the types, subtypes and strains of circulating viruses, and the level of protective antibodies in the general population. Although influenza epidemics may also occur regularly in tropical and subtropical regions, the disease patterns in these regions are less well established.

Timing of regional influenza activity

The timing of influenza activity around the world varies depending upon the climate of each region. In temperate climates, the onset and peak of influenza activity may vary substantially from one influenza season to the next but activity generally begins to increase in late autumn. In temperate regions of the northern hemisphere, influenza viruses are frequently isolated in the autumn, winter and spring. Periods of peak influenza activity typically occur between December and March and last for 6–8 weeks. In temperate regions of the southern hemisphere, influenza activity typically peaks in May to September. Although temperate regions of the world experience such seasonal peaks in influenza activity, influenza viruses can be isolated sporadically throughout the year, usually associated with outbreaks in closed environments such as nursing homes and summer camps.

The timing of seasonal peaks in influenza activity in tropical and subtropical countries also varies by region, and in some areas more than one peak of activity may occur in the same year. For example, in Hong Kong SAR, peaks in influenza activity can be seen in February–March and again during July–August associated with the monsoon season. In Singapore, peaks in influenza type A activity during the period 1990–1994 were seen in November–January and June–July, while influenza type B viruses were generally most active during March–April, July and December. In Panama, peaks in activity have been recorded during May–August, and in Zambia during June–August. Such variability in influenza seasonal peaks in tropical and subtropical countries illustrates the importance of country-specific and regional epidemiological and virological data including decisions on timing of vaccination programmes. Influenza viruses in tropical and subtropical regions can circulate at low levels at any time of the year and can cause isolated cases of influenza as well as outbreaks outside the peak periods of activity.

Epidemiology of pandemic influenza

In addition to the annual seasonal epidemics of influenza seen in some regions, pandemics of influenza have occurred infrequently and at irregular intervals. In all age groups, influenza infection rates are generally higher during pandemics than during annual epidemics. As with epidemics, school-age children play an important role in the spread of pandemic influenza in the community. During the course of the 20th century three pandemics occurred:

- **1918–1919** – the "Spanish flu" A(H1N1) pandemic led to more than 40 million deaths worldwide (Palese, 2004). Nearly half of these deaths were among people 20–40 years of age, and case-fatality rates of 30% were reported among pregnant women.
- **1957–1958** – the "Asian flu" A(H2N2) pandemic was associated with a total excess mortality of more than 1 million deaths globally (Lipatov et al., 2004).
- **1968–1969** – despite the lack of well-established estimates, the global excess mortality caused by the "Hong Kong flu" A(H3N2) pandemic has been calculated at around 1 million (Lipatov et al., 2004).

In all cases, the pandemic spread throughout the world within a year of its initial detection. Outbreaks of the Asian flu were first reported in late February 1957 in China and spread to other parts of Asia by April–May. Quarantine efforts were not helpful in curtailing the spread. By June, outbreaks were reported among passengers and crew on board ships bound for ports in the United States and Europe. After the initial introduction of the virus, small outbreaks in closed populations were detected in June and July and community-wide outbreaks were detected during August. School openings in the United States and Canada were followed by widespread dissemination of the virus in those countries during September, and peak mortality occurred by late October. In all three pandemics, people aged under 65 years accounted for a larger proportion of deaths in the United States than is usually seen in a typical influenza season.

The spread of **pandemic (H1N1) 2009** was even more rapid due to the high mobility and interconnectedness of 21st century societies. Within 6 weeks of first being described, it had affected all six WHO regions resulting in the declaration of a pandemic. Once again schools appeared to play an important role in the amplification of virus transmission. In previously unaffected countries, the virus was often detected first in schools where it caused intense outbreaks before spreading to the larger community. The appearance of the virus in the northern hemisphere during the summer months resulted in multiple intense localized outbreaks involving large communities. It arrived in the southern hemisphere at the start of the winter and transmission in those areas resembled an intense influenza season with a rapid rise in cases spread throughout the country and a rapid drop-off of cases within 10–12 weeks. Outbreaks were associated with increases in outpatient visits and a significant number of severely ill patients requiring intensive care and mechanical ventilation for severe viral pneumonia. The overall rates of severe disease, however, were considerably lower than those recorded for the pandemic of 1918. The rapidity with which the pandemic (H1N1) 2009 virus spread highlighted the need for timely and effective surveillance systems to detect emerging viruses with pandemic potential, and the need for standard platforms for data sharing and dissemination.

Influenza disease and its impact

Influenza is an acute respiratory disease caused by influenza type A or B viruses. For seasonal influenza, the incubation period ranges from 1 to 4 days. In infected adults, peak virus shedding usually occurs from 1 day before onset of symptoms to 3 days after onset, but may last longer in young children. The typical features of seasonal influenza include abrupt onset of fever and respiratory symptoms such as cough (usually non-productive), sore throat and coryza, as well as systemic symptoms such as headache, muscle ache and fatigue. The clinical severity of infection can range from asymptomatic infection to primary viral pneumonia and death. Acute illness generally lasts about 1 week, although malaise and cough may continue for 2 weeks or longer. Common complications of influenza infection include secondary bacterial pneumonia and exacerbation of underlying chronic health conditions; and otitis media in children. Uncommon complications include myositis, myocarditis, toxic-shock syndrome and Reye syndrome which is generally associated with the use of aspirin and other salicylate-containing medications in children and adolescents with influenza-like illness (ILI).

The symptoms of pandemic (H1N1) 2009 influenza in people were similar to those of seasonal influenza and included fever, cough, sore throat, body aches, headache, chills and fatigue. There were also reports of diarrhoea and vomiting associated with pandemic (H1N1) 2009 influenza. Illness in most cases was mild but there were cases of severe disease requiring hospitalization and a number of deaths. People at higher risk included those with underlying chronic diseases, immunosuppressed individuals, pregnant women and young children. Other at-risk groups included the morbidly obese and in some cases healthy individuals aged 15–50 years. Initial data from pandemic (H1N1) 2009 indicated that the incubation period for illness related to this virus was similar to that for seasonal influenza viruses. It is anticipated that the vius will persist in the population, with antigenic drift, as has occurred for earlier pandemic viruses.

Unlike influenza viruses that have achieved ongoing transmission in humans, the sporadic human infections with avian A(H5N1) viruses are far more severe with high mortality. Initial symptoms include a high fever (usually with a temperature higher than 38 °C) and other influenza-like symptoms. Diarrhoea, vomiting, abdominal pain, chest pain, and bleeding from the nose and gums have also been reported as early symptoms in some patients. Watery diarrhoea without blood appears to be more common in H5N1 influenza than in normal seasonal influenza. The disease often manifests as a rapid progression of pneumonia with respiratory failure ensuing over several days. It also appears that the incubation period in humans may be longer for avian (H5N1) viruses, ranging from 2 to 8 days, and possibly as long as 17 days.

Impact of influenza

Increases in the circulation of influenza viruses are associated with increases in acute respiratory illnesses, physician visits, hospitalizations and deaths. In general, rates of primary influenza illness are highest among school-age children (exceeding 30% in some years) and are lower among adults. During non-pandemic years, influenza infection rates among adults are estimated to generally range from 1% to 15%.

Morbidity

Although the highest rates of seasonal influenza-related illness occur among school-age children, the highest rates of associated hospitalizations occur among:

- children under 2 years of age;
- people of any age with certain chronic medical conditions (including chronic heart disease, lung disease such as asthma, diabetes, renal failure or immunocompromising conditions);
- those aged 65 years or older; and
- pregnant women.

For example, one study from the United States (Izurieta et al., 2000) estimated that healthy children under 2 years of age have 12 times the risk of influenza-related hospitalization as healthy children aged 5–17 years. Influenza-associated hospitalization rates are also higher among those with chronic medical conditions than among otherwise healthy people of the same age group. At both extremes of the age spectrum, however, rates of influenza-related hospitalization are elevated, even among those without chronic medical conditions. Rates of seasonal influenza-associated hospitalization are highest for people aged 85 years or older. The rates are lower for children and young adults, but children younger than 5 years old have hospitalization rates similar to people aged 50–64 years. Pregnant women also appear to be at increased risk of complications from influenza. One study of pregnant women enrolled in the Tennessee Medicaid Program in the

United States (Hartert et al., 2003) demonstrated that the relative risk of hospitalization for selected cardiorespiratory conditions increased from 1.4 during weeks 14–20 of gestation to 4.7 during weeks 37–42 compared to women who were 1–6 months postpartum. The risk of hospitalization during the influenza season in women in their third trimester of pregnancy (250 per 100 000 pregnant women) was comparable with the risk for non-pregnant women who had high-risk medical conditions.

During the influenza seasons 1990–1991 to 2000–2001 in the United States, it is estimated that an average of over 200 000 people were hospitalized for influenza-associated respiratory and circulatory illnesses each year (Thompson et al., 2004). Hospitalization rates have been found to be generally higher in seasons in which influenza A(H3N2) viruses have predominated as opposed to influenza type B or influenza A(H1N1) viruses (Simonsen et al., 2000). In one study of people discharged from hospitals in the United States during the 1979–1980 to 2000–2001 influenza seasons, the average estimated rates of influenza-related hospitalization were: 99 per 100 000 people during A(H3N2)-predominant years; 81.4 per 100 000 during B-predominant years; and 55.9 per 100 000 during A(H1N1)-predominant years (Thompson et al., 2004).

Mortality

Influenza-related deaths can result from pneumonia or from the exacerbation of existing cardiopulmonary conditions or other chronic conditions. Studies have estimated that in the United States the number of influenza-related pulmonary and circulatory deaths increased from 19 000 per influenza season from 1979–1980 to 1989–1990 to approximately 36 000 per season from 1989–1990 to 2002–2003 (Thompson et al., 2003). This increase might be partly due to the ageing of the population, and to the fact that the predominant virus during the majority of the influenza seasons from 1990 to 2003 was influenza A(H3N2) – a virus subtype associated with higher mortality. Studies in Europe have demonstrated rates of influenza-related death similar to those seen in the United States (Zucs et al., 2005).

In the United States, more than 90% of seasonal influenza-related deaths currently occur among people aged 65 years or older. The risk of influenza-related death increases with age and with the presence of underlying chronic conditions, particularly diabetes, and cardiovascular and pulmonary conditions. For example, one study (Barker & Mullooly, 1982) found the risk of death from seasonal influenza among people aged 45 years or older to be 39 times higher among those with 1 high-risk condition and 202 times higher among people with 2 or more high-risk conditions, compared with those with no high-risk conditions. An increased risk of influenza-related death among pregnant women was first observed during the 1918–1919 and 1957–1958 pandemics. As with hospitalization rates, influenza-related deaths have generally been higher in those years in which influenza A(H3N2) viruses have predominated.

1.B
Influenza control

Influenza vaccines

Annual vaccination is the primary means of reducing the impact of seasonal influenza. Vaccination is associated with reductions in:

- influenza-related respiratory illness and physician visits among all age groups;
- hospitalizations and deaths among people at high risk;
- otitis media among children; and
- work absenteeism levels among adults.

Currently, seasonal influenza vaccines contain a trivalent mixture of inactivated strains of the influenza viruses likely to circulate during the next influenza season. Because influenza viruses are constantly changing, the seasonal influenza vaccines are updated and administered annually to provide the necessary protection. Typically one or two of the three virus strains used in the vaccine will be changed each year.

Live attenuated and inactivated seasonal influenza vaccines

Live attenuated seasonal influenza vaccines[1] have been in development for over 50 years in Russia and the United States. Live vaccine has been used for some years in Russia and in 2003 one such vaccine was licensed for use in the United States for healthy people aged 2–49 years. Healthy people may choose this vaccine if they wish to avoid influenza infection themselves or if they are in close contact with people at high risk of developing serious complications from influenza infection. The live, trivalent vaccine is intranasally administered and is composed of virus strains that are:

- attenuated – producing mild or no signs or symptoms related to influenza infection;
- temperature-sensitive – a property that limits their ability to replicate at 38–39 °C thus restricting efficient viral replication in human lower airways; and
- cold-adapted – the vaccine viruses replicate efficiently at 25 °C, a temperature that restricts replication of various wild-type viruses.

Inactivated seasonal influenza vaccines are similar in many respects to live attenuated influenza vaccines. They both contain similar strains of influenza viruses representative of the recommended strains. The virus strains for both types of vaccine are selected annually, and one or more of these may be changed based on the results of global influenza surveillance and the emergence of new strains. Viruses for both types of vaccine are tra-

---

[1] A full discussion of live attenuated influenza vaccines can be found in Smith et al., 2006.

ditionally grown in eggs but can also be grown in cell cultures. As with live attenuated influenza vaccines, inactivated influenza vaccines also need to be administered annually to provide optimal protection against infection.

The major differences between inactivated and live attenuated influenza vaccines are:

- inactivated vaccines contain killed virus components, whereas live attenuated vaccine contains viruses still capable of limited replication;
- inactivated vaccine is administered intramuscularly whereas live attenuated vaccine is administered intranasally; and
- inactivated vaccine is approved for use in any person aged 6 months or older, whereas in the United States live attenuated vaccine is only approved for use in healthy people aged 2–49 years. In the Russian Federation, live attenuated influenza vaccines are licensed for immunizing children aged 3–15 years and adults.

Antiviral drugs for influenza

Antiviral drugs for controlling and preventing influenza are an adjunct to the use of influenza vaccines. In general, four influenza antiviral agents are licensed or partially licensed in various countries:

- amantadine;
- rimantadine;
- zanamivir and
- oseltamivir.

Controlled clinical trials have demonstrated that all four drugs reduce the duration of symptoms when used for the treatment of influenza infection and can also prevent illness when used for chemoprophylaxis. The costs, routes of administration, adverse effects, contraindications and potential for antiviral resistance differ among the four drugs. There are insufficient data on the use of any of these drugs during pregnancy.

Based on their chemical properties and spectrum of activity against influenza viruses, the drugs can be classified into two categories, **adamantane derivatives** (amantadine and rimantadine) and **neuraminidase (NA) inhibitors** (zanamivir and oseltamivir). A meta-analysis and systematic review of published studies (Burch et al., 2009) has concluded that when used for treatment, both the adamantane derivatives (**BOX 1.B-1**) and the NA inhibitors (**BOX 1.B-2**) are effective in reducing the duration of symptoms of influenza type A infection by approximately one day compared with placebo administration. Furthermore, clinical studies have reported that the NA inhibitors generally result in fewer serious side-effects (compared with placebo administration) than have been reported for the adamantane derivatives.

BOX 1.B-1

Adamantane derivatives

Amantadine and rimantadine are chemically related drugs that specifically inhibit the replication of influenza type A viruses – but not influenza type B viruses.

■ **Antiviral activity** – the mechanism of action of adamantane derivatives is not completely understood, but it is believed that they interfere with the function of the transmembrane domain of the M2 protein of influenza type A viruses. They also interfere with influenza type A virus assembly during viral replication. As a result they prevent the release of infectious influenza A viral particles from the host cell.

■ **Effectiveness** – controlled studies have found that when administered within 48 hours of the onset of illness, both drugs are effective in decreasing viral shedding and in reducing the duration of illness of influenza type A infections by approximately one day compared with placebo administration. The recommended duration of treatment is usually 5 days. When used for chemoprophylaxis, both drugs are approximately 70–90% effective in preventing the symptoms of illness resulting from influenza type A infection. When used for treatment neither appears to affect the ability of the body to develop antibodies to influenza A and antibodies can also be produced during prophylaxis should viral exposure occur while taking the drug. The efficacy and effectiveness of both drugs in preventing the complications of influenza type A are unknown.

■ **Side-effects** – adverse gastrointestinal and central nervous system effects have been reported during controlled chemoprophylaxis studies in healthy adults and elderly nursing-home residents. The chemoprophylactic use of both drugs has been associated with central nervous system toxicity effects such as light-headedness, difficulty concentrating, nervousness, insomnia and seizures in patients with pre-existing seizure disorders. Rimantadine use has been associated with fewer central nervous system side-effects than amantadine. Amantadine is teratogenic and embryo toxic in animals. Rimantadine has not been found to be mutagenic. The safety of amantadine and rimantadine use during pregnancy has not however been established.

■ **Antiviral resistance** – the use of adamantane derivatives for treatment has been associated with the rapid selection and development of resistant virus strains. Drug-resistant virus strains can then spread to the contacts of treated individuals, including those receiving chemoprophylaxis. Because the mechanism of resistance is the same for both adamantane derivatives, influenza type A viruses resistant to one are also resistant to the other. However, resistance to adamantane derivatives does not affect the susceptibility of viruses to NA inhibitors.

BOX 1.B-2

Neuraminidase (NA) inhibitors

Zanamivir and oseltamivir are chemically related members of a new class of antiviral drugs active against both influenza type A and B viruses. Zanamivir is an orally inhaled powdered, whereas oseltamivir is given as an orally administered capsule or oral suspension. Other forms of delivery of these drugs (e.g. intravenous) and additional NA-inhibitors are currently being developed.

■ **Antiviral activity** – the mechanism of action of both drugs involves blocking the active site of the viral enzyme NA which is common to both influenza type A and B viruses. This results in viral aggregation at the infected host cell surface and the prevention of progeny virus release from the cell.

■ **Effectiveness** – when treatment is initiated within 48 hours of the onset of illness, both drugs are effective in decreasing viral shedding and reducing the duration of symptoms of influenza infection by approximately one day, compared with placebo administration. The recommended duration of treatment is 5 days. Controlled studies have demonstrated the efficacy of both drugs, when used prophylactically, in preventing the symptoms of illness resulting from influenza infection in adults and adolescents compared with placebo administration. Oseltamivir is indicated for the treatment and chemoprophylaxis of influenza type A and B in adults and children aged one year and older. Zanamivir is indicated for the treatment and chemoprophylaxis of influenza type A and B in adults and children aged >5 years.

■ **Side-effects** – oseltamivir use has been associated with nausea and vomiting during controlled treatment studies compared with placebo administration. Nausea, diarrhoea, dizziness, headache and cough have been reported during zanamivir treatment but the frequencies of adverse events were similar to those seen with orally inhaled powder placebo. Few serious central nervous system adverse effects have been reported for these drugs. Zanamivir is not generally recommended for use in people with underlying respiratory disease because of the risk of precipitating bronchospasm. Serious respiratory adverse events resulting from zanamivir use have been reported in people with chronic pulmonary disease and in healthy adults. Data are limited regarding the potential use of NA inhibitors to treat influenza during pregnancy.

■ **Antiviral resistance** – in 2008 a high proportion of seasonal H1N1 viruses were found to have resistance to oseltamivir but were still sensitive to zanamivir. Influenza type A(H3N2) and B viruses remain sensitive to both NA inhibitors. The majority of pandemic (H1N1) influenza viruses characterized in 2009 were sensitive to oseltamivir but a small number of resistant viruses were detected. All pandemic (H1N1) 2009 viruses analysed in 2009 were sensitive to zanamivir. In vitro studies have found that resistance to NA inhibitors does not affect the susceptibility of viruses to adamantane derivatives.

1.C
Influenza surveillance

WHO Global Influenza Surveillance Network

In 1952, following discussions on the creation of an international network of influenza laboratories that could provide annual recommendations on the composition of influenza vaccines, WHO initiated the Global Influenza Surveillance Network (GISN). As of 2010, the network consisted of:

- 136 National Influenza Centres (NICs)[1] in 106 Member States;
- 4 WHO Collaborating Centres (WHOCCs) for Reference and Research on Influenza, 1 WHOCC for Surveillance, Epidemiology and Control of Influenza, and 1 WHOCC for Studies on the Ecology of Influenza in Animals;[2] and
- 4 key national reference laboratories involved in WHO influenza vaccine virus selection and development.

In response to public health needs arising from avian influenza A(H5N1) infection in humans and the need to strengthen influenza pandemic preparedness, the WHO H5 Reference Laboratory Network was established in 2004 as an ad hoc component of the GISN (**FIGURE 1.C-1**). This network includes WHOCCs and other laboratories with internationally recognized expertise in avian influenza.[3]

Since its establishment, the major objective of the GISN has been to provide the detailed virological information required by WHO to make annual recommendations on the composition of influenza vaccines for the northern and southern hemispheres. In addition, the GISN serves as the primary global alert mechanism for detecting the emergence of novel influenza viruses that could cause an influenza pandemic. This latter role has become increasingly important.

As part of its range of activities and functions[4] the designated NIC within each country receives or collects clinical specimens from the national laboratory network in order to conduct preliminary analyses. When reporting the results of virological surveillance, NICs are advised to follow the procedures outlined in current WHO guidance.[5] NICs also send representative seasonal virus isolates to at least one of the five WHOCCs located in Atlanta (United States), Beijing (China), London (United Kingdom), Melbourne (Australia), and

---

[1] www.who.int/csr/disease/influenza/centres/en/index.html
[2] www.who.int/csr/disease/influenza/collabcentres/en/index.html
[3] www.who.int/csr/disease/avian_influenza/guidelines/referencelabs/en/
[4] www.who.int/csr/disease/avian_influenza/guidelines/RoleNICsMay07/en/index.html – pending revision.
[5] *Human infection with pandemic (H1N1) 2009 virus: updated interim WHO guidance on global surveillance.* Geneva, World Health Organization. 10 July 2009. www.who.int/csr/resources/publications/swineflu/interim_guidance/en/index.html

FIGURE 1.C-1
The WHO Global Influenza Surveillance Network (GISN)

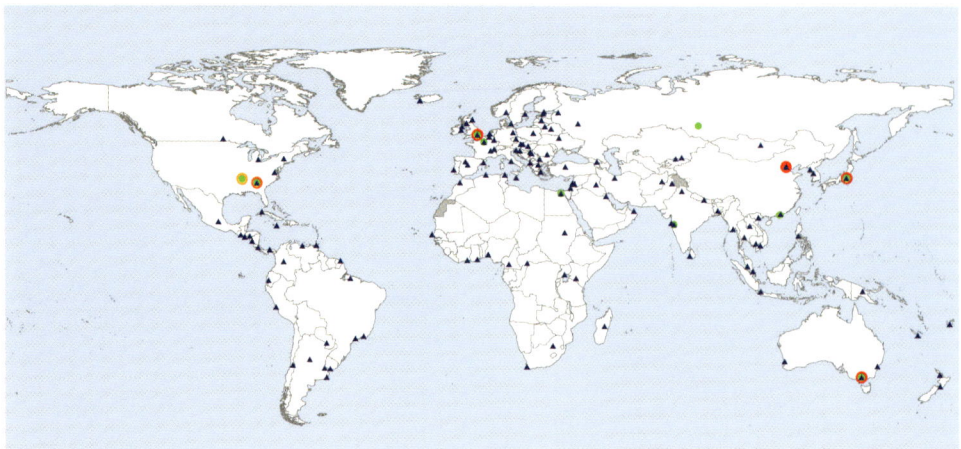

▲ National Influenza Centres
● H5 Reference Laboratories
● WHO Collaborating Centre for Studies on the Ecology of Influenza in Animals
● WHO Collaborating Centre for Surveillance, Epidemiology and Control of Influenza
● WHO Collaborating Centre for Reference and Research on Influenza

Tokyo (Japan). Influenza viruses of animal origin such as avian H5N1 can also be sent to the WHOCC in Memphis (United States). The WHOCCs conduct more advanced antigenic and genetic analyses, the results of which form the basis of the WHO annual recommendations on the composition of influenza vaccines. They also prepare and distribute updated influenza reagent kits to all NICs and other collaborating laboratories each year. These kits, which include reference antisera and control antigens, are needed to identify circulating influenza A(H3N2), A(H1N1) and B viruses, and for serological testing. Kits specific for influenza A(H5N1) viruses are also available on request from the WHOCCs.

Networking and information resources
FluNet

FluNet[1] is an Internet-based communications tool developed by WHO in 1997 to support and coordinate national influenza surveillance and to facilitate global reporting. A new version of FluNet was launched in February 2004 that included more-powerful functions such as mapping and chart-making capabilities. Upon request by e-mail (gisn@who.int) NICs can obtain permission to forward weekly reports to FluNet during the influenza season. An updated summary of global influenza activity based mainly on the reports made by NICs to WHO via FluNet is then produced.[2] At the national level the following information is also made available to the public:

■ number of specimens processed per week;
■ number of isolates obtained by subtype (i.e. A(H1), A(H3), A(H5), pandemic (H1N1) 2009, A(not subtyped) and B);
■ national level of influenza-like illness (ILI) activity;

[1] www.who.int/flunet
[2] www.who.int/csr/disease/influenza/update/en/index.html

- a brief weekly report of the overall estimated influenza activity in a country; and
- contact information for the NICs.

Vaccine recommendations

The annual WHO recommendations on the composition of influenza vaccines are normally published on the WHO web site[1] the day after the relevant WHO consultation. In the case of vaccine strain selection for the northern hemisphere winter the consultation is held in February, and for the southern hemisphere winter in September–October. In tropical areas the local epidemiology of influenza may determine the timing of vaccination and, therefore, the choice of preferred vaccine formulation.

Weekly Epidemiological Record

Summaries of global influenza activity are published frequently in the *Weekly Epidemiological Record*.[2] The WHO influenza vaccine composition recommendations are also normally published here 2–3 weeks after the WHO consultations are completed.

WHO Influenza Information Platform

To facilitate communication among the various networks, a restricted-access web site[3] for different user groups has been set up. Access is provided only to approved groups which can then post and view documents. For example, detailed antigenic and genetic information as well as antigenic cartographic analyses presented at WHO information meetings following the WHO annual consultation on influenza vaccine composition can be viewed on the site by NIC staff.

Information resources

- Information on the WHO GISN is available at:
  www.who.int/csr/disease/influenza/surveillance/en/index.html
- Information on pandemic (H1N1) 2009 is available at:
  www.who.int/csr/disease/swineflu/en/index.html
- Information on the global response to human cases of H5N1 avian influenza and on monitoring the corresponding threat of an influenza pandemic is available at:
  www.who.int/csr/disease/avian_influenza/en/index.html
- Other information about influenza and the WHO Global Influenza Programme (GIP) is available at:
  www.who.int/influenza

The precise organization and implementation of mechanisms to ensure the effective surveillance of influenza disease in humans and its virological characteristics will depend upon national and regional characteristics and on the available resources and priorities of individual countries. However, there are a number of key principles that underlie both **disease** and **virological** surveillance, both of which are essential in:

- establishing the epidemiological patterns of influenza;
- understanding the risk factors related to severe influenza;
- assessing the burden of influenza;

---

[1] www.who.int/csr/disease/influenza/vaccinerecommendations1/en/index.html
[2] www.who.int/wer/en/
[3] http://ezcollab.who.int/Default.aspx

- updating the composition of seasonal influenza vaccines;
- assessing and monitoring the antiviral susceptibility of circulating seasonal influenza strains;
- detecting and identifying novel influenza viruses that have the potential to cause a pandemic;
- assisting in prototype pandemic vaccine development and assessing and monitoring the antiviral susceptibility of emerging strains.

Disease surveillance
Assessment of influenza activity levels

Monitoring the patterns of influenza epidemics is essential for the yearly planning of prevention and response activities; for identifying groups at high risk of complications; and for estimating the health and economic burden of influenza. A variety of clinical outcomes can be monitored, but the present global standard is to monitor both severe acute respiratory infection (SARI) and influenza-like illness (ILI). Ideally, a surveillance system would therefore include both SARI (or severe hospitalized cases) and ILI (or milder outpatient-managed cases) in order to understand and describe the entire spectrum of influenza-related disease.

Influenza disease surveillance (for both SARI and ILI) is generally based upon a limited number of **sentinel sites** strategically located so as to represent the diverse climatic, sociological and ethnic diversity in a country. Information on health-care visits for respiratory illness can be obtained and reported from such sites, which can include the offices of adult, family or paediatric physicians, and other outpatient or hospital-associated clinics such as university student health clinics or emergency departments. Sites can be selected in such a way that population catchment areas can be estimated to facilitate the estimation of disease burden. The systematic selection of cases for sampling – rather than "convenience" selection – with accompanying collection of epidemiological and clinical data will provide representative data that can identify the population at risk for severe disease, the clinical spectrum of illness related to influenza, and other epidemiological characteristics. These data can be invaluable in planning influenza control measures. The surveillance of clinically diagnosed SARI and ILI should also be linked to virological surveillance (see below).

Analysis of **hospital discharge data** for pneumonia and influenza can also be useful in tracking and characterizing severe illness related to influenza. Unless the medical records are fully computerized, such data may not be available on a real-time basis. In such situations, an analysis of hospitalizations can more easily be carried out as a retrospective study rather than as a weekly analysis. Alternatively, hospital admission diagnosis or chief complaint data may be used rather than discharge diagnoses to facilitate incidence monitoring. Regardless of the actual data used, surveillance will be greatly facilitated by the availability of computerized medical records. However, it should be noted that both admission and discharge data are prone to coding biases and coding errors.

Other sources of data that may reflect influenza activity (and can therefore be monitored for surveillance) include school or workplace **absenteeism**, sales of over-the-counter or prescription **medicines** used to treat influenza, and increases in **ambulance calls**. However, each data source has significant weaknesses and may reflect factors that are unrelated to influenza activity. In particular, work or school absenteeism is highly non-specific, and trends in absenteeism should therefore be interpreted with caution. Nonetheless, if data are readily available they can be used to complement other more specific outcomes.

Reporting of influenza activity levels

In addition to FluNet there are a number of other influenza disease surveillance and reporting systems currently in use worldwide. Selected examples of these systems are shown in **BOXES 1.C-1–1.C-4**. As with FluNet, both EuroFlu (the European system) and the United States surveillance systems report estimated levels of overall influenza activity. In both FluNet and EuroFlu, estimated levels of activity are reported for countries (or regions within a country). In the United States, estimated levels of activity are reported for the country, and sometimes for surveillance regions or states. While each of these systems uses standard definitions to report activity levels, it is important to note that the surveillance and reporting methods (and the precise definitions of activity levels) may vary from country to country and even from state to state. As a result, data collection and interpretation are not currently standardized, and involve subjective decisions. Nonetheless, this does provide very useful information often reflecting local interpretation that may otherwise be lacking. A more unified approach would however be desirable and would provide reports that were more directly comparable.

Participating countries in FluNet report their influenza activity levels as:

- **no activity** – no influenza viral isolates or clinical signs of influenza activity;
- **sporadic activity** – an isolated case of ILI or laboratory/culture-confirmed influenza cases in a limited area;
- **local activity** – ILI activity above baseline values with laboratory-confirmed influenza cases in a limited area;
- **regional activity** – outbreaks of ILI or laboratory-confirmed influenza in one or more regions, with the number of cases comprising less than 50% of the country's total population; and
- **widespread activity** – outbreaks of ILI or laboratory-confirmed influenza in one or more regions, with the number of cases comprising 50% or more of the country's population.

Monitoring the **number of deaths** related to the clinical outcome of influenza infection can provide accurate denominator-based information on the severity of influenza in a community. For example, deaths in which pneumonia or influenza are mentioned on the death certificate can be recorded to monitor the trends and impact of an influenza season. Information on the impact of influenza can help the public health community to communicate the serious consequences of influenza and to justify the implementation of preventive measures such as vaccination.

As data on deaths often lag behind morbidity data, the former are often less useful than virological or disease surveillance data in the detection of outbreaks. Moreover, mortality reporting systems can be costly. However, death surveillance is extremely useful for monitoring the severity of influenza seasons and for documenting the seriousness of the health impact of influenza. The concurrent availability of laboratory-based virological data to aid in the interpretation of mortality data is essential.

> ### BOX 1.C-1
>
> **China**
>
> A nationwide influenza surveillance network has been in place since 2000. Its functions include ILI monitoring, severe respiratory disease surveillance, outbreak surveillance and virological surveillance. By mid-2009, 197 sentinel hospitals and 84 influenza laboratories (covering national to prefecture levels) had been enrolled in the network.
>
> Respiratory specimens are collected from all sentinel hospitals, with at least 5 specimens collected from each hospital every week during normal influenza seasons and 15 during epidemics. Specimen collection from ILI cases must occur within 3 days after onset of symptoms and only from individuals who have not received antiviral drug treatment. Specimens are generally sent to influenza laboratories within 48 hours of collection and are kept at 4 °C; if this is not the case, specimens are stored at -70 °C.
>
> The daily number of ILI visits and the daily total of outpatients in sentinel hospitals are recorded and reported in five age groups (0–4 years; 5–14 years; 15–24 years; 25–59 years; and 60 years and older). All information related to epidemiological and virological surveillance is reported through the National Influenza/Avian Influenza in Humans Surveillance Information System. In southern China, influenza surveillance is carried out all-year round, while in northern China it is conducted from October to March.
>
> Outbreaks of influenza or ILI are reported by disease-control institutions at all levels to the national health authority through the Public Health Emergency Report and Management System. Specimens are collected and tested using either rapid tests or virus-isolation techniques in the reporting institutions, and the results forwarded through the National Influenza/Avian Influenza in Humans Surveillance Information System. All virus isolates and/or positive specimens are shipped to the Beijing WHOCC for prompt confirmation and further characterization.
>
> The WHOCC also conducts further antigenic and genetic analysis in support of the public health activities of WHO – including the issuing of WHO vaccine composition recommendations and vaccine virus development.

Virological surveillance

All national and international influenza surveillance systems – including those for monitoring clinical disease – depend fundamentally upon virological surveillance. Within countries, the NIC serves as the focal point for coordinating influenza virological surveillance. Some primarily collect specimens directly while others primarily receive virus isolates from other influenza laboratories. NICs also provide technical advice to national policy-makers and serve as the key point of contact between WHO and national authorities on questions related to influenza surveillance and the provision of influenza virus isolates to WHOCCs. This role includes immediate notification of the detection of unusual viruses and of influenza outbreaks to national authorities and WHO GISN. As with disease surveillance, approaches to virological surveillance differ by country and by region.

The following key components of the virological surveillance of influenza are discussed in detail in **PART 2** (**SECTIONS 2.A–2.L**) of this manual:

BOX 1.C-2

Europe

In the WHO European Region, clinicians, epidemiologists and virologists in the 53 Member States constitute the network reporting to EuroFlu (www.euroflu.org/index.php). The laboratory network consists of WHO-recognized NICs and the Community Network of Reference Laboratories for Human Influenza in Europe (www.euroflu.org/html/lb_description.html). The main goal of this regional surveillance system is to contribute to a reduction in morbidity and mortality due to influenza in Europe. Euroflu replaced the European Influenza Surveillance Scheme that was created in 1996.

Reporting countries have at least one national sentinel surveillance network for collecting information on the number of ILI or ARI cases (or both). The case definitions can differ slightly from country to country. Most countries also collect information on the age of ill people. In countries where the population under surveillance is known (e.g. from physician patient lists) or can be calculated, population-based rates are estimated and reported. In addition to describing the geographical distribution of influenza viruses, a second variable is incorporated to describe the intensity of influenza activity compared with historical data on clinical influenza activity outside of epidemic periods (baseline level). This variable is divided into the following categories:

- **low intensity** – influenza activity does not exceed the baseline level;
- **medium intensity** – influenza activity is at the expected level;
- **high intensity** – influenza activity is higher than expected; and
- **very high intensity** – influenza activity is particularly severe.

Sentinel physicians are also asked to take nasal and/or throat swabs from a sample of patients with ILI or ARI. In some national sentinel surveillance networks, blood samples are also collected. More recently, the WHO Regional Office for Europe has issued new surveillance guidelines that include SARI as part of the surveillance strategy.

Countries are currently working to establish inpatient surveillance to compliment their existing ILI surveillance. As part of this, the NICs also report influenza test results from physicians who are not part of the sentinel surveillance network and these data are compared with those received through the network. These additional data sources include inpatient facilities, nursing homes and clinics. It is anticipated that there will sometimes be differences between viruses collected from patients in hospitals and those collected from outpatients (e.g. in the proportion of viruses of a particular subtype).

2.A Collection, storage and transport of specimens

Clinical specimens that are to be tested for influenza viruses can be collected either as part of routine patient care (through sentinel surveillance) or during outbreak investigations. The successful isolation of an influenza virus depends upon the prompt collection of high-quality specimens, the rapid transportation of specimens to the testing laboratory, and appropriate transport and storage conditions prior to testing. Ideally, respiratory specimens and acute-phase serological specimens should be collected within 3 days of the onset of clinical symptoms.

> ### BOX 1.C-3
>
> **Kenya**
>
> In 2006, the Kenya Ministry of Health established national influenza surveillance through a sentinel network of 10 hospitals – seven provincial hospitals, a large referral hospital in Nairobi, and hospitals in two refugee camps. Surveillance officers at each site screen patients for both SARI and ILI. For every SARI patient, a short questionnaire with demographic and clinical information is completed, and respiratory specimens (swabs) are collected. Specimens are sent to the NIC – a laboratory connected to the Kenya Medical Research Institute in Nairobi – where they are tested for influenza by real-time reverse transcription polymerase chain reaction (RT-PCR). Positive samples are cultured in Kenya, and isolates sent to a WHOCC for further characterization. Monthly reports are distributed to stakeholders describing the levels of SARI, ILI and influenza activity.

2.B Processing of clinical specimens for virus isolation

where good-quality clinical specimens are available, virus isolation is a highly sensitive and very useful procedure for the diagnosis of viral infection. One important advantage of virus isolation is that it amplifies the amount of virus in the original specimen, thus producing a sufficient quantity for further antigenic and genetic characterization, and for drug-susceptibility testing if required.

2.C Virus isolation in cell culture

The isolation of viruses in cell cultures is increasingly becoming the gold standard for virus diagnosis. However a laboratory must maintain several cell lines to allow for the detection of a variety of respiratory pathogens. Since standard virus-isolation procedures take several days before results are available they are usually of limited use in clinical settings for the prompt diagnosis of influenza.

2.D Virus isolation in embryonated chicken eggs

In recent years, the use of cell cultures has surpassed the use of embryonated eggs to isolate and culture influenza viruses. However, only viruses grown in embryonated eggs can be used as seed viruses for the production of the majority of influenza vaccines. For this reason, laboratories that have the capability to isolate influenza viruses in eggs are encouraged to maintain this capacity.

2.E Identification of the haemagglutinin subtype of viral isolates by haemagglutination inhibition testing

The haemagglutination inhibition (HAI) test is an extremely reliable assay for typing, subtyping and further determining the antigenic characteristics of influenza viral isolates provided that the reference antisera used contain antibodies to currently circulating viruses. The antisera used are based on antigen preparations derived from either the wild-type strain or a high-growth reassortant made using the wild-type strain or an antigenically equivalent strain.

BOX 1.C-4

United States

In the United States, over 2000 sites are enrolled in an influenza sentinel surveillance reporting system. Each week from October to May, approximately 2400 sentinel health-care providers report on the number of patient visits and on the number of those visits that were for ILI by age group (0–4 years; 5–24 years; 25–64 years; and 65 years and older). These data are used to calculate national weekly ILI visits as a percentage of all patient-care visits – as well as separate percentages for each of the nine influenza surveillance regions in the country.

Because the patient population served by each participating health-care provider is unknown, population-based rates are not estimated. However, the United States also has a population-based network of hospital reporting sites in 12 major metropolitan areas that reports the rates of severe hospitalized influenza. This system initially reported just on children (under the age of 17 years) but was expanded in 2005–2006 to include all age groups. The output of this system is the population-based rate of hospitalized influenza.

In the United States, the following three data sources are used to monitor influenza-related mortality:

- the 122 Cities Mortality Reporting System (122 MRS) – a timely reporting system that monitors the weekly percentage of deaths related to pneumonia or influenza in 122 American cities (http://aspe.hhs.gov/DATACNCL/DataDir/cdc2.htm);

- all paediatric deaths related to laboratory-confirmed influenza – these are now nationally reportable deaths; and

- periodic analyses using national vital statistics to estimate the overall numbers of deaths from influenza.

Estimates of the number of deaths from influenza reflect the concept of "excess" deaths. In essence, if the proportion of deaths related to pneumonia or influenza in a given week (as reported through the 122 MRS) exceeds the expected baseline percentage of such deaths for that week by a statistically significant amount, then these deaths are said to exceed the epidemic threshold. If influenza viruses are in general circulation in the area at that time, then such excess deaths can be attributed to influenza.

Health-care providers also collect nasal and throat swabs for virus isolation from a subset of patients with ILI. Testing is then generally performed by the state public health laboratory, and the virus isolation data entered into the national virological surveillance system. A combined network of approximately 120 laboratories located in state or local health departments, universities or hospitals collaborate with WHO and with the National Respiratory and Enteric Virus Surveillance System. Information and subsets of viral isolates are sent to the Centers for Disease Control and Prevention (CDC) in Atlanta (which is a WHOCC). The isolates then undergo complete antigenic and genetic characterization. During the influenza season, the CDC sends WHO a weekly summary report of the results via FluNet.

The disadvantages of the HAI test include the need to remove nonspecific inhibitors of haemagglutination that occur naturally in sera; the need to standardize reference and test antigens each time a test is performed; and the need for specialized expertise in reading the results of the test. Nevertheless, the HAI test remains the assay of choice for global influenza surveillance and for determining the antigenic characteristics of influenza viral isolates.

2.F Serological diagnosis of influenza by haemagglutination inhibition testing

Diagnosing influenza by virus isolation in cell culture definitively identifies the infecting strain and is usually more rapid than serological diagnosis. However, serological diagnosis is an important approach when clinical specimens are unobtainable or when a laboratory does not have the resources required for virus isolation. Serological methods such as the HAI test are essential for many epidemiological and immunological studies and for evaluation of the antibody response following vaccination. Serological methods are also very useful in situations where identification of the virus is not feasible (e.g. after viral shedding has stopped).

Demonstration of an acute influenza infection using serology requires a significant increase in antibody titres (i.e. 4-fold or greater) between acute-phase and convalescent-phase serum samples. The demonstration of such a significant increase may establish the diagnosis of a recent infection even when attempts to detect the virus are negative.

2.G Serological diagnosis of influenza by microneutralization assay

Serological methods such as the HAI test rarely yield an early diagnosis of acute influenza virus infection. Although conventional neutralization tests for influenza viruses (based on the inhibition of cytopathogenic effect formation in MDCK cell culture) are laborious and rather slow, a microneutralization assay using microtitre plates in combination with an ELISA to detect virus-infected cells can yield results within two days. The microneutralization assay is a highly sensitive and specific assay for detecting virus-specific neutralizing antibodies to influenza viruses in human and animal sera, potentially including the detection of human antibodies to avian subtypes. Testing can be carried out quickly once a novel virus is identified and often before purified viral proteins become available for use in other assays.

2.H Identification of neuraminidase subtype by neuraminidase assay and neuraminidase inhibition test

There are two basic forms of assay for influenza virus neuraminidase (NA) based on the use of different substrate molecules, a long-standing assay based on the use of a large substrate such as fetuin and newer assays which utilise small substrate molecules. Although the older assay is more cumbersome and difficult to perform it remains useful because antibody to the neuraminidase will block access to a large but not necessarily to a small substrate molecule. The fetuin-based method is used to determine the potency of the viral NA and thus the standardized NA dose for use in the NA inhibition (NAI) test. Once determined, the standardized dose is added to serial dilutions of test antisera, negative control serum and reference anti-NA serum. Any inhibitory effect of the sera on NA activity can then be determined and the NAI titre calculated.

2.I Molecular identification of influenza isolates

The direct molecular identification of influenza isolates is a rapid and powerful technique. The reverse-transcription polymerase chain reaction (RT-PCR) allows template viral RNA to be reverse transcribed producing complementary DNA (cDNA) which can then be amplified and detected. This method can be used directly on clinical samples and the rapid nature of the results can greatly facilitate investigation of outbreaks of respiratory illness. For example, genetic analysis of influenza virus genes (especially the HA and NA genes) can be used to identify an unknown influenza virus when the antigenic characteristics cannot be defined. Genetic analyses also can be used to monitor the evolution of influenza viruses and to determine the degree of relatedness between viruses from different geographical areas and those collected at different times of the year.

2.J Virus identification by immunofluorescence antibody staining

Immunofluorescence antibody (IFA) staining of virus-infected cells in original clinical specimens and field isolates is a rapid and sensitive method for diagnosing respiratory and other viral infections. During recent years, monoclonal antibodies against several clinically important respiratory viruses have become commercially available and have been thoroughly evaluated in many laboratories. It is preferable for IFA staining to be performed on isolates rather than original clinical specimens as this allows any virus that is present to first be amplified, and if required used in other studies. However, where rapid diagnosis is needed, this procedure is often carried out on clinical specimens. Because commercially available rapid tests for diagnosing influenza infection differ with regard to the type of specimen required, as well as their complexity, specificity and sensitivity, WHO recommends that such assays should be used in conjunction with other laboratory tests.[1]

2.K Use of neuraminidase inhibition assays to determine the susceptibility of influenza viruses to antiviral drugs

The emergence of marked resistance to oseltamivir among seasonal A(H1N1) viruses during late 2007 to early 2008 has made it imperative to conduct NA inhibitor susceptibility surveillance among circulating influenza viruses worldwide. A number of different methods have been developed for this purpose, and the two procedures presented in this section have been based upon the Centers for Disease Control and Prevention (CDC) chemiluminescent NAI assay, and the National Institute for Medical Research (NIMR) NAI MUNANA assay. Whichever method is selected, a local risk assessment should be conducted and a suitable level of biosafety containment used – especially for viruses with pandemic potential.

---

[1] www.who.int/csr/disease/avian_influenza/guidelines/rapid_testing/en/index.html

PART 2
The laboratory diagnosis and virological surveillance of influenza

2.A Collection, storage and transport of specimens

Clinical specimens that are to be tested for influenza viruses can be collected either as part of routine patient care (through sentinel surveillance) or during outbreak investigations. Successful influenza virus diagnosis depends largely upon the quality of the specimen and the conditions under which it is stored and transported prior to laboratory processing. Specimens for the isolation of influenza viruses in cell culture and for the direct detection of viral antigens or nucleic acids should ideally be collected within 3 days of the onset of clinical symptoms.

An acute-phase serum specimen (3–5 ml whole blood) should be taken promptly after the onset of clinical symptoms – and no later than 7 days afterwards. A convalescent-phase serum specimen should subsequently be collected 2–4 weeks later. Single serum specimens cannot reliably be used for the diagnosis of influenza virus infection, except for a presumptive diagnosis during an outbreak situation (see **SECTION 2.F**).

Materials required[1]

Equipment

Vacuum source	Centrifuge (low speed)

Supplies

Sputum/mucus trap with 10 French gauge (FG) catheter **Vygon – catalogue (cat.) no. 542.10**	Centrifuge tubes (conical, 15 ml) **BD Biosciences (Falcon) – cat. no. 352097**
Transport system, e.g. Viral Culturette System **Fisher Scientific – cat. no. 14-910-46**	Transfer pipettes **Samco – cat. no. 336-200**
Cotton-tipped applicator **Copan Diagnostics – cat. no. 165K501**	Polyester fibre-tipped applicator **BD Biosciences (Falcon) – cat. no. 2069**
Filter (0.22 µm pore-size membrane) **Millipore – cat. no. SLGS 033 SS**	Collection vials (optional)
Beaker or Petri dish	

---

[1] In this and all subsequent sections, the mention of specific companies or of certain manufacturers' products does not imply that they are endorsed or recommended by the World Health Organization in preference to others of a similar nature that are not mentioned. The expiry dates of all products should be checked before use.

Buffers, reagents[1] and media

Washing fluid (e.g. physiological saline (0.85% NaCl); see instructions below)	Dulbecco's Modified Eagle Medium (D-MEM) high glucose (1x), liquid, with L-glutamine, without sodium pyruvate **Invitrogen – cat. no. 11965-092**
Transport medium (e.g. Hanks' Balanced Salt Solution) **Invitrogen – cat. no. 14175-095**	Gentamicin reagent solution (50mg/ml); liquid **Invitrogen – cat. no. 15750-078**
Tryptose-phosphate broth **Difco – cat. no. 260300**	Veal infusion broth **Sigma – cat. no. V5262**
Bovine albumin fraction V (7.5%) **Invitrogen – cat. no. 15260-037**	Amphotericin B, 250 µg/ml **Invitrogen – cat. no. 15290-018**
Gelatin **Difco – cat. no. 214340**	Water (distilled and sterile)
Water (distilled and deionized)	

Preparation of solutions

Physiological saline (0.85% NaCl)

a. Prepare a 20x stock solution by dissolving 170 g NaCl in deionized distilled water to a total volume of 1 litre.
b. Sterilize by autoclaving.
c. To prepare physiological saline (0.85% NaCl) add 50 ml 20x stock solution to 950 ml of deionized distilled water.
d. Sterilize by autoclaving.
e. Store opened physiological saline at 4 °C for no longer than 3 weeks.

Washing fluid

Physiological saline, Hanks' balanced salt solution or cell culture medium – without antibiotics and proteins – can all be used as washing fluids.

Transport medium

The following formulation of transport medium is recommended for use in the specimen-collection procedures outlined below:

a. Add 10 g veal infusion broth and 2 g bovine albumin fraction V (7.5%) to sterile distilled water to a volume of 400 ml.
b. Add 0.8 ml gentamicin sulfate solution (50 mg/ml) and 3.2 ml amphotericin B (250 µg/ml).
c. Sterilize by filtration using a 0.22 µm pore-size membrane.

---

[1] Analytical grade reagents should be used for all procedures described in this manual.

Specimen-collection procedures

Barrier protection should be used by all staff collecting samples from patients

For the diagnosis of viral infections of the ***upper*** respiratory tract, the following specimens are both suitable and easily collected:

- **nasal swab** – a dry cotton (or polyester-fibre) tipped swab is inserted into the nostril parallel to the palate and left in place for a few seconds before being slowly withdrawn using a rotating motion. Specimens from both nostrils are obtained with the same swab. The tip of the swab is placed into a collection vial or directly into a 15 ml conical centrifuge tube containing 2–3 ml transport medium and the applicator stick is broken off.
- **throat swab** – both tonsils and the posterior pharynx are swabbed vigorously and the swab placed into a collection vial or directly into a 15 ml conical centrifuge tube containing 2–3 ml transport medium and the applicator stick is broken off.
- **combined nasal and throat swab** – nasal and throat swabs are taken as described above and then placed into the same vial or tube containing transport medium.
- **nasopharyngeal aspirate** – nasopharyngeal secretions are aspirated through a catheter connected to a sputum/mucus trap and fitted to a vacuum source. The catheter is inserted into one nostril parallel to the palate. The vacuum is then applied and the catheter is slowly withdrawn with a rotating motion. Mucus from the other nostril is collected with the same catheter in a similar manner. After mucus has been collected from both nostrils, the catheter is flushed with 3 ml transport medium.
- **nasal wash** – the patient sits in a comfortable position with the head tilted slightly backward and is advised to keep the pharynx closed by saying the letter K ("kay") while washing fluid (usually physiological saline) is applied. Using a transfer pipette, 1.0–1.5 ml washing fluid is applied to one nostril at a time. The patient then tilts the head forward and lets the fluid flow into a beaker or Petri dish. The process should be repeated alternately in each nostril until a total of 10–15 ml washing fluid has been used. The washing fluid is then divided into approximately 3 ml aliquots and each aliquot diluted 1:2 in transport medium.
- **throat wash** – the patient gargles with 10 ml washing fluid. The fluid is collected into a beaker or Petri dish and diluted 1:2 in transport medium.

If clinically indicated one of the following invasive procedures can be performed to obtain specimens for the diagnosis of viral infection of the ***lower*** respiratory tract:

- transtracheal aspiration;
- bronchoalveolar lavage; or
- lung biopsy.

For the serological diagnosis of influenza, serum can be collected as below:

- **serum** – draw whole blood by syringe or into a plain vacutainer tube. Collect the blood in a hard plastic or glass tube; blood will not clot in soft plastic. Allow the blood to clot for 30 minutes to 1 hour at room temperature. "Rim" the clot with a Pasteur pipette (separate it from the walls of the collection tube to allow clot contraction). Place the rimmed specimen in the refrigerator overnight. Pipette the serum off of the clot and place into a clean test tube. Clarify by centrifugation at 2000–3000 rpm for 10 minutes. Remove clarified serum from the pellet and store in suitable containers.

Storage and transport of specimens

Specimens should be collected, stored and transported using a suitable medium. Several transport systems are commercially available (e.g. the Viral Culturette System) that have proven to be satisfactory for the recovery of a wide variety of viruses. In addition to the recommended formulation above, Hanks' balanced salt solution, cell culture medium, tryptose-phosphate broth and veal infusion broth are all commonly used transport media. Whichever of these is used should be supplemented with protein (e.g. bovine albumin fraction V (7.5%) or gelatin) to a concentration of 0.5–1% to stabilize the viruses. The addition of antibiotics and antimycotics is also advised to help prevent microbial growth.

Specimens intended for the direct detection of viral antigens by immunofluorescence staining of infected cells should be kept on ice and processed within 1–2 hours of collection.

Specimens for virus isolation should be placed at 4 °C immediately after collection and promptly transported to the laboratory. Processed specimens should be inoculated into susceptible cell cultures as soon as possible. If the specimens cannot be processed within 48 hours, they should be kept frozen at or below -70 °C – ideally in liquid nitrogen. In order to prevent loss of infectivity, repeated freezing and thawing must be avoided.

Sera may be stored at 4 °C for approximately 1 week but for periods longer than this should be frozen at -20 °C.

The transportation of specimens should comply with current WHO guidance[1] on the transporting of infectious substances. Receiving laboratories in other countries should be notified in advance of specimens being sent to allow them time to arrange an import licence.

---

[1] www.who.int/csr/resources/publications/swineflu/storage_transport/en/index.html

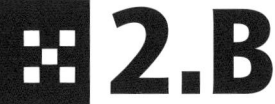

2.B
Processing of clinical specimens for virus isolation

Virus isolation is generally a highly sensitive and very useful procedure for the diagnosis of viral infection when clinical specimens are of good quality and have been collected promptly – ideally within 3 days of the onset of clinical symptoms. One important advantage of virus isolation is that it amplifies the amount of virus in the original specimen, thus producing a sufficient quantity for further antigenic and genetic characterization, and for drug-susceptibility testing if required.

Materials required

Equipment

| Vortex mixer | Centrifuge (low speed) |

Supplies

| Collection vials (optional) | Glass beads (small) |
| Centrifuge tubes (conical, 15 ml)
BD Biosciences (Falcon) – cat. no. 352097 | |

Reagents

| Gentamicin reagent solution (50 mg/ml); liquid
Invitrogen – cat. no. 15750-078 | |

Protocol for processing specimens

Nasal, throat, and combined nasal and throat swabs

1. Vigorously agitate the collection vial or centrifuge tube containing the swab and transport medium on a vortex mixer. Release the fluid by grasping the end of the swab-stick and squeezing the tip against the inner wall of the vial or tube.
2. Remove the swab from the vial or tube and add 0.2 ml gentamicin solution per ml of transport medium to give a final concentration of 10 mg/ml.
3. Leave at room temperature for 15 minutes.
4. Transfer the specimen to a centrifuge tube (if not collected directly into one) and centrifuge at 1000 rpm for 5 minutes.
5. Remove supernatant and use 200 µl for virus isolation (see **SECTION 2.C**), and store any remaining supernatant at between -70 °C and -80 °C.

Nasopharyngeal aspirates, and nasal and throat washings

1. Break up mucus clumps by adding small glass beads to the specimen and homogenizing vigorously on a vortex mixer.

2. Add 0.2 ml gentamicin solution per ml of specimen to give a final concentration of 10 mg/ml.
3. Leave at room temperature for 15 minutes.
4. Transfer the specimen to a centrifuge tube (if not collected directly into one) and centrifuge at 1000 rpm for 10 minutes to remove extraneous materials.
5. Remove supernatant and use 200 µl for virus isolation (see **SECTION 2.C**), and store any remaining supernatant at between -70 °C and -80 °C.

Precautions

In addition to the proper safety procedures that must be observed when handling all influenza viruses (see **ANNEX I**) special precautions should be taken when working with clinical specimens and with laboratory-adapted or reference influenza virus strains.

Some laboratories prepare their own laboratory-adapted control influenza viruses from stock viruses for use as positive controls. In addition, laboratories frequently use commercially available influenza reference viruses for their quality assurance programmes. Because such viruses are selected for their optimal growth properties, laboratory-adapted and reference influenza virus strains pose a serious risk of cross-contamination with clinical specimens.

It is therefore extremely important that all laboratory-adapted controls are prepared, tested and stored well in advance of the influenza season. If laboratory-adapted control viruses must be replenished during the influenza season, this should be done on days when clinical material is not being inoculated. Likewise, quality assurance tests with commercial reference viruses should be performed outside the influenza season or on days when clinical material is not being inoculated. Acceptable laboratory practice always requires that known viruses and unknown materials must be worked with at different times and preferably in separate biosafety cabinets or rooms. If the latter is not possible, thorough clean-down of cabinets should be undertaken between the different activities and the cabinet allowed to run for at least 30 minutes.

In summary the following practices should always be adhered to:

- Be aware of the potential for clinical specimens to become contaminated with laboratory-adapted strains or reference viruses.
- Never process clinical specimens for virus isolation at the same time as laboratory-adapted or reference influenza strains.
- Never process clinical specimens from humans in the same laboratory specimens taken from swine or birds.
- Never store viral isolates at -20 °C as this will result in the loss of virus viability due to freeze/thaw cycles.
- Maintain cell lines and prepare cultures for use in virus isolation in a dedicated virus-free cabinet preferably in a dedicated laboratory.

Since influenza viruses are continuously evolving, older strains are antigenically distinct from currently circulating strains. Because laboratory-adapted viruses and commercial reference viruses are prepared using older strains, complete antigenic analysis by haemagglutination inhibition (HAI) testing using selected ferret antisera and DNA sequencing can be performed to determine if an isolate has been inadvertently contaminated.

2.C Virus isolation in cell culture

Although the isolation of viruses in cell cultures (with subsequent identification of the virus by immunological or genetic techniques) has traditionally been considered the gold standard for virus diagnosis, there are several factors that must be taken into consideration. Each of the currently available mammalian cell lines supports the replication of only a limited number of clinically important respiratory viruses. A laboratory must therefore maintain several cell lines in order to detect a variety of respiratory pathogens. On the basis of clinical and epidemiological information, the appropriate cell lines to be inoculated will have to be selected for each specimen. Madin-Darby canine kidney (MDCK) cells are typically the preferred cell line in which to culture influenza viruses.

Standard isolation procedures require an average of 4–5 days before results are available, making them of limited use to the clinician. Rapid culture assays that use immunological methods to detect viral antigens in cell culture have however become available – the results of these assays can be obtained in 18–40 hours.

The following protocol for the isolation of influenza viruses in cell culture (using MDCK cells) allows for virus identification by immunofluorescence antibody staining and provides a virus isolate for further analysis. Daily readings of both cytopathic effect and harvest data should be recorded (see **ANNEX II**).

Materials required

Equipment

Incubator (34–37 °C)	Centrifuge (low speed)
Microscope (inverted)	

Supplies

Tissue culture flasks (T-75 canted neck) **Corning – cat. no. 430720**	Tissue culture flasks (T-25 canted neck) **Corning – cat. no. 430168**
Filter (0.22 μm pore-size membrane) **Millipore – cat. no. SLGS 033 SS**	Pipettes (1 ml) **BD Biosciences (Falcon) – cat. no. 357503**
Centrifuge tubes (conical, 15 ml) **BD Biosciences (Falcon) – cat. no. 352097**	Pipettes (10 ml) **BD Biosciences (Falcon) – cat. no. 357530**

Cells, buffers, reagents and media

MDCK cells American Type Culture Collection, **ATCC CCL 34**	Fetal bovine serum (FBS); irradiated **Cambrex – cat. no. 14-471F**
D-MEM high glucose (1x); liquid; with L-glutamine; without sodium pyruvate **Invitrogen – cat. no. 11965-092**	Trypsin-ethylenediaminetetraacetic acid (trypsin-EDTA) (0.05% trypsin; 0.53 mM EDTA · 4Na) **Invitrogen – cat. no. 25300-054**
Penicillin-streptomycin (stock solution contains 10 000 U/ml penicillin; and 10 000 µg/ml streptomycin sulfate) **Invitrogen – cat. no. 15140-148**	Trypsin L-1-tosylamide-2-phenylethyl chloromethyl ketone (TPCK-trypsin); treated (type XIII from bovine pancreas) **Sigma – cat. no. T1426**
HEPES (N-2-hydroxyethylpiperazine-N'-2-ethane sulfonic acid) Buffer (1 M stock solution) **Invitrogen – cat. no. 15630-080**	Gentamicin reagent solution (50 mg/ml); liquid **Invitrogen – cat. no. 15750-078**
Bovine albumin fraction V (7.5%) **Invitrogen – cat. no. 15260-037**	Glycerol
Gelatin **Difco – cat. no. 214340**	

Preparation of media and solutions

Complete D-MEM

To 470 ml D-MEM add:

Reagent	Volume	Final concentration
Penicillin-streptomycin	5.0 ml	100 U/ml penicillin;100 µg/ml streptomycin
Bovine albumin fraction V (7.5%)	12.5 ml	0.2%
HEPES buffer	12.5 ml	25 mM

D-MEM medium for cell growth

To 450 ml complete D-MEM (prepared as above) add:

Reagent	Volume	Final concentration
FBS	50 ml	10%

D-MEM medium for virus growth

To 500 ml complete D-MEM (prepared as above) add:

Reagent	Volume	Final concentration
TPCK-trypsin solution (2 mg/ml)	0.5 ml	2 µg/ml

TPCK-trypsin stock solution (2 mg/ml)

a. Dissolve 20 mg TPCK-trypsin in 10 ml complete D-MEM medium for virus growth. Phosphate Buffered Saline (PBS) may be used as an alternative to the D-MEM medium: see 2-E for recipe). Filter through a 0.22 µm pore-size membrane.

b. Store in aliquots at -20 °C.

Preparing an MDCK cell suspension

The procedure described below for preparing an MDCK cell suspension is for use with confluent T-25 flasks. If cell culture flasks of other sizes are used, the volumes must be adjusted correspondingly. Once the procedure is complete, one T-25 flask with a confluent monolayer of MDCK cells will contain approximately 10^7 cells.

1. Add 5 ml of trypsin-EDTA (pre-warmed to 37 °C) to each of the T-25 flasks containing the cell sheets and gently rock the flask for 1 minute. Remove trypsin-EDTA with a pipette. Typsin-Phospate Buffered Saline can be used as an alternative to the trypsin-EDTA in steps 1 and 2.
2. Add another 5 ml trypsin-EDTA and gently rock flask for 1 minute. Remove trypsin-EDTA with a pipette.
3. Add 1 ml trypsin-EDTA and distribute over entire cell sheet – incubate flask at 37 °C until all cells detach from plastic surface (5–10 minutes). The flask may need shaking or hitting to detach cells.
4. Add 1 ml FBS to inactivate remaining trypsin.
5. Add 8 ml complete D-MEM. Pipette up and down gently to break up cell clumps.
6. Transfer the 10 ml mixture to 90 ml D-MEM medium for cell growth. This cell suspension contains approximately 10^5 cells per ml.
7. Add 6 ml (600 000 cells) of this cell suspension to an appropriate number of T-25 flasks. The remaining cell suspension can be used to seed T-75 flasks for cell passage. Usually 5 ml cell suspension added to 20 ml D-MEM medium for cell growth provides an adequate number of cells for obtaining a confluent monolayer in several days.
8. Incubate flasks at 37 °C.

Quality control

Over a number of passages, MDCK cells can lose their susceptibility to respiratory viruses. For this reason, the laboratory should keep a stock of frozen cells at a low passage level. At the beginning of each influenza season, an aliquot of such low-passage cells should be thawed and used during the entire season providing that the cells remain healthy and this does not exceed 25 consecutive passages or 3 months. Cell lines should be free of Mycoplasma contamination.

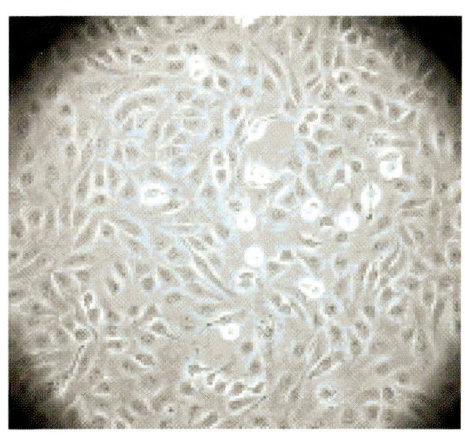

FIGURE 2.C-1
Uninfected Madin-Darby canine kidney cells

Inoculation of cell cultures

All the following steps must be performed in a class-II biosafety cabinet to avoid the contamination of cells.

Preparation of cells

1. Check that the cells are healthy and in a monolayer using a microscope at 40x magnification (see **FIGURE 2.C-1**).
2. Discard the D-MEM medium for cell growth from the flasks and wash

the cells 3 times with 6 ml complete D-MEM or Phosphate Buffered Saline.

Inoculation of cells

1. Remove medium from flask with a pipette.
2. Inoculate 200 µl of each processed specimen (see **SECTION 2.B**) into a T-25 flask using pipettes.
3. Allow inoculum to adsorb for 30 minutes at 37 °C.
4. Add 6 ml D-MEM medium for virus growth (containing 2 µg/ml of TPCK-trypsin) to the flask.
5. Incubate at 35 °C and observebserve daily for the cytopathic effect shown in **FIGURE 2.C-2**.

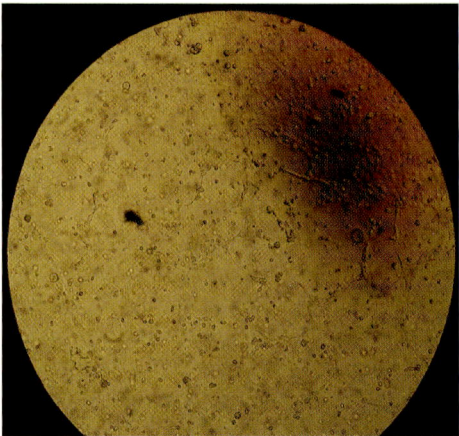

FIGURE 2.C-2
Cytopathic effect typical of influenza infection in Madin-Darby canine kidney cells

Harvesting virus

1. Harvest the virus if 3+ or 4+ (75–100%) cytopathic effect is observed by collecting the supernatant fluid and adding 0.5% stabilizer such as glycerol, gelatin or bovine albumin fraction V (7.5%). Harvest by day 6 or 7 even if no cytopathic effect is observed.
2. Perform a haemagglutination test (see **SECTION 2.E**) and store the viral isolate at 4 °C. If there is no haemagglutination, passage cells 1 or 2 more times before reporting an inability to recover virus from the specimen.
3. If necessary, centrifuge the tubes at 3000 rpm for 5 minutes to remove excess cells. Identify the isolate by haemagglutination inhibition (HAI) testing (see **SECTION 2.E**) and store the isolate at -70 °C within 2 days of harvesting.

Note that in some seasons the success of isolation can be increased by a 'blind' passage of a sample of the supernatant from a flask that has not shown evidence of cytopathic effect or presence of HA.

2.D
Virus isolation and passage in embryonated chicken eggs

In recent years, the use of cell cultures has surpassed the use of embryonated eggs to isolate and culture influenza viruses. However, only viruses grown in embryonated eggs can be used as seed viruses for the production of the majority of influenza vaccines. As a result, the trend towards the use of cell culture has decreased the availability of suitable vaccine viruses. For this reason, laboratories that have the capability to isolate influenza viruses in eggs are encouraged to maintain this capacity.

All the steps described below must be performed in a class-II biosafety cabinet to avoid contamination. A record should be kept of inoculation and harvest data (see **ANNEX III**).

Materials required

Equipment

Egg candler	Sharps safety container
Incubator (preferably humidified)	Centrifuge (low speed)

Supplies

Embryonated chicken eggs (9-11 days old)	All-purpose non-toxic glue or paraffin wax
70% ethanol **Fisher Scientific - cat. no. S73985**	Centrifuge tubes (conical, 15 ml) **BD Biosciences (Falcon) - cat. no. 352097**
Needle; 22 gauge; 1½ inch (3.8 cm) **BD Biosciences (Falcon) - cat. no. 305156**	Pipettes (10 ml) **BD Biosciences (Falcon) - cat. no. 357530**
Tuberculin syringe (1 ml) **Monoject - cat. no. 501400**	Forceps (sterile) **Fisher Scientific - cat. no. 08-887**
Egg hole punch (hole can also be made with large syringe, cannula and rubber stopper)	Egg trays

Candling and inoculation of eggs

Candling of eggs

1. Examine eggs with an egg candler.
2. Discard any eggs that are infertile, have cracks, are underdeveloped or that appear to have a very porous shell.

Inoculation of eggs

1. Place eggs into egg trays with the blunt end up, and label eggs with a specific identification number (allocating 3 eggs for each specimen).
2. Wipe the blunt end of each egg with 70% ethanol and punch a small hole in the shell over the air sac.
3. Aspirate 0.6 ml of processed specimen into a tuberculin syringe with a 22 gauge, 1½ inch needle.
4. Holding the egg up to the candler, locate the embryo. Insert the needle into the hole in the shell and, using a short stabbing motion, pierce the amniotic membrane and inoculate 100 μl of the specimen into the amniotic cavity. Withdraw the needle by about ½ inch (1.25 cm) and inoculate 100 μl of the specimen into the allantoic cavity. Remove the needle.
5. Inoculate the two other eggs allocated to the specimen in the same manner with the same syringe and needle to give a total of 3 eggs inoculated per specimen.
6. Discard the syringe and needle, placing them in a proper safety container.
7. Seal the hole punched in the eggs with a drop of glue or wax.
8. Incubate the eggs as follows – for H5N1 viruses (24–30 hours at 37 °C); for H3N2 and H1N1 viruses (2 days at 37 °C); and for influenza B viruses (3 days at 35 °C).

Note: H5N1 inoculation must be done under BSL3 conditions.

Harvesting virus from inoculated chicken eggs

1. Chill eggs at 4 °C overnight before harvesting. An alternate method is to chill at -20 °C for 30 minutes – however, overnight at 4 °C is preferable.
2. Label one centrifuge tube (15 ml) with the specimen number for one egg. Clean the blunt end of each egg with 70% ethanol.
3. With sterile forceps, break the shell over the air sac and push aside the allantoic membrane with the forceps. Using a 10 ml pipette, aspirate the allantoic fluid and place it in the labelled centrifuge tube. Then using a syringe and needle, pierce the amniotic sac and remove as much amniotic fluid as possible. Place the amniotic fluid in a separate tube – however, because of the small volume of this fluid obtained from each egg, it is usually necessary to combine the amniotic fluid obtained from all 3 of the eggs allocated to each specimen.
4. Perform a haemagglutination test (see **SECTION 2.E**) and store the viral isolate at 4 °C. If there is no haemagglutination, passage the specimen in allantoic and amniotic fluid twice more before reporting an inability to recover virus from the specimen.
5. If necessary, centrifuge the tubes at 2000 rpm for 10 minutes to remove excess blood and tissues. Identify the isolate by HAI testing (see **SECTION 2.E**) and store the isolate at -70 °C within 2 days of harvest.

Passaging isolates and reference viruses in the allantoic cavity

Allantoic passage can be used for the further adaption of viruses that have given positive haemagglutination in the amniotic or allantoic fluid harvests. Amplification of egg-adapted virus stocks may be performed as follows:

1. Place eggs into egg trays with the blunt end up, and label eggs with a specific identification number (allocating 3 eggs for each specimen).
2. Wipe the blunt end of each egg with 70% ethanol and punch a small hole in the shell over the air sac.
3. Aspirate 0.6 ml of processed specimen into tuberculin syringe with a 22 gauge, 1½ inch needle.
4. Via the hole inoculate 0.2 ml of virus suspension. When the needle is fully inserted it should penetrate directly into the allantoic sac fluid. Usually 2–3 eggs are inoculated per specimen. Eggs are generally incubated at 33–35 °C for 2–3 days.
5. Following incubation chill as above, harvest allantoic fluid and test for haemagglutination.

2.E Identification of the haemagglutinin subtype of viral isolates by haemagglutination inhibition testing

The haemagglutination inhibition (HAI) test was originally described by Hirst (1942) and then later modified by Salk (1944). This traditional method for identifying influenza isolates takes advantage of the tendency of the haemagglutinin (HA) protein of influenza viruses to bind to red blood cells (RBCs) causing them to agglutinate. When antibodies against a specific influenza HA protein bind to the antigenic sites on the HA protein, these sites become blocked and therefore unavailable for binding with RBCs. The subsequent inhibition of haemagglutination is the basis for the HAI test.

Currently, the HAI test is performed using microtitre plates. A standardized quantity of HA antigen is mixed with serially diluted antiserum, and RBCs are then added to assess the degree of binding of the antibody to the HA molecule.

The HAI test is extremely reliable provided that the reference antisera contain antibodies to currently circulating viruses. The antisera used are based on antigen preparations derived from either the wild-type strain or a high-growth reassortant made using the wild-type strain or an antigenically equivalent strain. In the case of seasonal influenza, the antisera are newly prepared each year against the vaccine strains that are the prototypes for strains circulating at the time.

The disadvantages of the HAI test include the need to remove nonspecific inhibitors of haemagglutination that occur naturally in sera; the need to standardize reference and test antigens each time a test is performed; and the need for specialized expertise in reading the results of the test. Nevertheless, the HAI test remains the assay of choice for global influenza surveillance and for determining the antigenic characteristics of influenza viral isolates.

Materials required
WHO Influenza Reagent Kit

The following protocol is specific to the reagents supplied by CDC Atlanta. Note that different reagents are available (e.g. through the WHO CC Melbourne) which have different characteristics for which the protocol supplied with that kit should be followed.

The kit is prepared and distributed each year to participating WHO collaborating laboratories. It contains reagents for the identification of influenza A(H1N1), A(H3N2) and B viral isolates; as well as reagents for serological diagnosis.

Reference antisera for the identification of viral isolates are prepared either in sheep by multiple intramuscular injections with purified HA or in chickens by intravenous inoculation with virus grown in embryonated eggs. Control antigens consist of infected allantoic fluid inactivated by beta-propiolactone. The antigen preparations are derived from either the wild-type vaccine strain or a high-growth reassortant made using the wild-type strain or an antigenically equivalent strain.

The following reagents are provided:

Influenza A reagents for identification of viral isolates and serological diagnosis:
— influenza A(H1N1) control antigen
— influenza A(H3N2) control antigen
— influenza A(H1N1) reference antiserum
— influenza A(H3N2) reference antiserum

Influenza B reagents for identification of viral isolates:[1]
— influenza B control antigen (B/Yamagata/16/88 lineage)
— influenza B control antigen (B/Victoria/02/87 lineage)
— influenza B reference antiserum (B/Yamagata/16/88 lineage)
— influenza B reference antiserum (B/Victoria/02/87 lineage)

Influenza B reagents for serological diagnosis only:
— ether-treated influenza B control antigen (B/Yamagata/16/88 lineage)
— ether-treated influenza B control antigen (B/Victoria/02/87 lineage)

Other reagents:
— negative control serum
— receptor destroying enzyme (RDE)

Equipment

Water-bath (37 °C)	Centrifuge (low speed)
Water-bath (56 °C)	Laboratory shaker (optional)

Supplies

Pipettes (1 ml) BD Biosciences (Falcon) – cat. no. 357503	Pipettes (10 ml) BD Biosciences (Falcon) – cat. no. 357530
Haemacytometer (double rule "bright line") Reichert – cat. no. 1490	Haemacytometer coverslips Reichert – cat. no. 1492
Pipetman (1–200 µl) Rainin – cat. no. P-200	Tips for Pipetman (sterile) Rainin – cat. no. RT-20
Multichannel pipetter Rainin – cat. no. L12-200	Tips for multichannel pipetter Rainin – cat. no. RT-L200F
Centrifuge tubes (conical, 15 ml) BD Biosciences (Falcon) – cat. no. 352097	Centrifuge tubes (conical, 50 ml) BD Biosciences (Falcon) – cat. no. 352070
Racks for 15 ml centrifuge tubes Fisher Scientific – cat. no. 14-793-12	Racks for 50 ml centrifuge tubes Fisher Scientific – cat. no. 14-793-3
Gauze squares Fisher Scientific – cat. no. 19-041-951	Cell counter (2-unit counter) Clay Adams – cat. no. 4314
96-well microtitre plates (V-shaped for use with chicken or turkey RBCs) Nunc – cat. no. 249570	96-well microtitre plates (U-shaped for use with human type O or guinea-pig RBCs) Corning Life Sciences – cat. no. 3798
Filter (0.22 µm) Millipore – cat. no. SLGS 033 SS	

---

[1] ***Two*** sets of influenza B reagents are currently distributed to distinguish viral isolates belonging to the B/Yamagata/16/88 lineage and the B/Victoria/02/87 lineage. This situation may change if one or the other lineage disappears from circulation.

Cells, buffers and other materials

RBCs (chicken, turkey, guinea-pig or human type O) in Alsever's solution (see below)	Phosphate-buffered saline (PBS); (0.01 M, pH 7.2); (see below)
Water (distilled)	Physiological saline (0.85% NaCl); (see below)
Water (distilled and deionized)	

Preparation of solutions

PBS (0.01 M, pH 7.2)

a. Prepare a 25x stock solution containing in 100 ml: 2.74 g Na_2HPO and 0.79 g $NaH_2PO_4 \cdot H_2O$.

b. To prepare 0.01 M PBS, mix and dissolve in distilled water to a total volume of 1 litre: 40 ml PBS 25x stock solution and 8.5 g NaCl.

c. After thorough mixing, check pH = 7.2 ± 0.1 – if necessary adjust pH with 1 N NaOH or 1 N HCl.

d. Autoclave or filter (using a 0.22 µm pore-size membrane) to sterilize.

e. Store opened 0.01 M PBS at 4 °C for no longer than 3 weeks.

Alsever's solution for collection and storage of RBCs

a. Weigh out and dissolve in deionized distilled water to a total volume of 1 litre:
  — 20.5 g dextrose
  — 8.0 g sodium citrate dihydrate ($Na_3C_6H_5O_7 \cdot 2H_2O$)
  — 4.2 g NaCl
  — 0.55 g citric acid ($C_6H_8O_7$)

b. After thorough mixing, check pH = 6.1 ± 0.1 – if necessary adjust pH with 1 N NaOH or 1 N HCl.

c. Sterilize by filtration through a 0.22 µm pore-size membrane.

Note: contamination is likely in this solution if it is not adequately sterilized.

Physiological saline (0.85% NaCl)

a. Prepare a 20x stock solution by dissolving 170 g NaCl in deionized distilled water to a total volume of 1 litre.

b. Sterilize by autoclaving.

c. To prepare physiological saline (0.85% NaCl) add 50ml 20x stock solution to 950 ml deionized distilled water.

d. Sterilize by autoclaving.

e. Store opened physiological saline at 4 °C for no longer than 3 weeks.

Standardization of RBCs

The following procedure is commonly used. The final concentration of chicken and turkey RBCs is 0.5%; and that of guinea-pig and human type O RBCs is 0.75%. **Note: a higher concentration of guinea-pig and human type O RBCs is desirable for the visualization of complete settling of RBCs**:

1. Blood should be collected into a suitable anti-clotting agent such as an equal volume of Alsevers solution or a blood collection tube containing an appropriate amount of Lithium Heparin. Where human type O cells are used these should be from individuals screened and shown free of blood-borne pathogens.
2. Filter approximately 5 ml blood through gauze into a 50 ml conical centrifuge tube.
3. Centrifuge at 1200 rpm for 10 minutes.
4. Aspirate the supernatant and buffy layer of white blood cells.
5. Add 50 ml PBS (pH 7.2). Mix gently by inversion.
6. Centrifuge at 1200 rpm for 5 minutes. Aspirate the supernatant.
7. Repeat the PBS wash twice. **Note: do not over wash the cells as this can lead to haemolysis**.
8. Resuspend RBCs to a final volume of 12 ml in a 15 ml conical centrifuge tube.
9. Centrifuge at 1200 rpm for 10 minutes.
10. Either estimate the volume of packed cells and dilute them with PBS to the appropriate concentration or determine the concentration with a haemacytometer and adjust accordingly, as described below.

Determination and adjustment of RBC concentration by counting cells using a haemacytometer

1. Prepare a 1:100 dilution by adding 0.5 ml RBC suspension (from step **9** above) to 49.5 ml PBS (pH 7.2).
2. Clean the haemacytometer thoroughly with 70% ethanol and dry with lens tissue or a soft lint-free cloth. Clean and dry the coverslip in the same way and press it gently onto the haemacytometer so that it adheres to and covers the counting area.
3. Transfer 10 µl onto the haemacytometer channel and allow the cells to spread throughout the unit, being careful not to overfill the channel. This is done by loading the Pipetman with the suspension and bringing it to the edge of the space immediately beneath the coverslip and injecting the mixture slowly until the chamber is full.
4. Count the cells in each of the 4 large corner quadrants of the unit (shown in bold in **FIGURE 2.E-1**). Each quadrant contains 16 small squares.
5. After counting, rinse the chamber and coverslip with 70% ethanol and dry.
6. Calculate the final volume of RBC suspension as follows:

    (i) Avian RBCs – final volume for a 0.5% suspension of avian RBCs =

    $$= \frac{\text{the number of cells counted} \times \text{volume from step } \mathbf{1}}{160}$$

    (ii) Mammalian RBCs – final volume for a 0.75% suspension of mammalian cells

    $$= \frac{\text{number of cells counted} \times \text{volume from step } \mathbf{1}}{240}$$

    Note: the above formulas were determined as follows:

    $$\text{Cell count/ml} = \frac{\text{total cell count} \times \text{dilution factor} \times 10^4}{\text{no. of squares counted}}$$

FIGURE 2.E-1
Counting cells using a haemacytometer

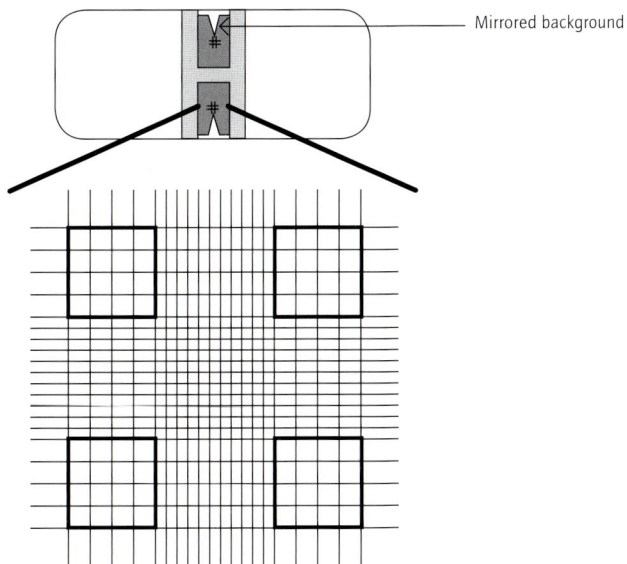

Treatment of reference antisera to inactivate nonspecific inhibitors of haemagglutination

The degree of sensitivity to nonspecific inhibitors of haemagglutination present in sera differs between influenza viral strains. The inactivation procedure below is specific for the RDE supplied in the WHO Influenza Reagent Kit. Since preparations of RDE vary, the RDE supplied in the kit is evaluated each year and the optimal procedure is determined using current influenza viral strains. This procedure is published in the kit insert and must be used with the accompanying kit reagents for accurate results. Any RDE from previous kits should not be used with the current kit reagents. Both the reference antisera and negative control serum should be treated.

1. Reconstitute the lyophilized reference antisera with distilled deionized water to the volume indicated on the label. Store the reconstituted antisera at -20 °C to -70 °C.
2. Reconstitute the RDE with the volume of physiological saline (0.85% NaCl) specified in the kit. Aliquot and store at -20 °C to -70 °C.
3. Add 3 volumes of RDE to 1 volume of serum (e.g. 0.9 ml RDE + 0.3 ml serum; **note: this volume of RDE is sufficient for testing 50–55 viral isolates)**.
4. Incubate overnight in a 37 °C water-bath.
5. Heat in a 56 °C water-bath for 30 minutes to inactivate any remaining RDE.
6. Allow sera to cool to room temperature. Add 6 volumes of physiological saline. The final dilution of sera is therefore 1:10 (e.g. 0.9 ml RDE + 0.3 ml serum + 1.8 ml physiological saline).

Detection of nonspecific agglutinins in treated sera

Nonspecific agglutinins must be removed from sera to prevent false negatives in the HAI test.

1. Choose the appropriate type of 96-well microtitre plate (see **TABLE 2.E-1**) and label as shown in **FIGURE 2.E-2**.[1]
2. Add 25 μl PBS (pH 7.2) to the first 6 wells in rows B to H (i.e. B1–B6; C1–C6; etc. up to H1–H6).
3. Add 50 μl PBS to the first well in column 6 (A6) for an RBC control.
4. Add 50 μl of each RDE-treated serum to the first 5 wells in row A (A1–A5).
5. Prepare serial 2-fold dilutions of the sera by transferring 25 μl from the first well of columns 1–6 to the successive wells in each column (i.e. A1 to B1; then B1 to C1; etc. up until G1 to H1). Discard the final 25 μl after row H.
6. Add 25 μl PBS to all wells (instead of antigen) in columns 1–6.
7. Add 50 μl standardized RBCs (see the standardization procedure for RBCs above) to all wells of columns 1–6.
8. Mix using a laboratory shaker or by manually agitating the plates thoroughly.
9. Incubate the plates at room temperature for the appropriate time by checking the RBC control for complete settling of the cells. A total of 30 minutes is usually required for chicken or turkey RBCs to settle and 60 minutes for guinea-pig or human type O RBCs (**TABLE 2.E-1**).
10. Record and interpret the results in accordance with **TABLE 2.E-1** and **FIGURE 2.E-3**.

If the RBCs settle completely in the wells in a column containing diluted serum, that serum is acceptable for use in the HAI test. The presence of nonspecific agglutinins will be evident by any haemagglutination of the RBCs by the serum. In this case, the serum must be adsorbed with RBCs as follows:

1. To one volume of packed RBCs in a centrifuge tube add 20 volumes of RDE-treated serum.
2. Mix thoroughly and incubate at 4 °C for 1 hour, mixing at intervals to resuspend the cells.

TABLE 2.E-1
Haemagglutination with different types of red blood cells (RBCs)

Characteristic	Type of RBC			
	Chicken	Turkey	Guinea-pig	Human type O
Concentration (%)	0.5	0.5	0.75	0.75
Type of microtitre plate	V	V	U	U
Incubation time at room temperature (minutes) after RBCs added	30	30	60	60
Appearance of control RBCs	Button[a]	Button[a]	Halo	Halo

[a] RBC pellet flows when plate is tilted.

---

[1] Throughout this manual, the wells of the microtitre plate designated A–H on the 3 inch (7.5cm) side are called **rows** and those designated 1–12 on the 5 inch (12.5 cm) side are called **columns**.

FIGURE 2.E-2
Schematic outline approach for the detection of nonspecific agglutinins in treated sera

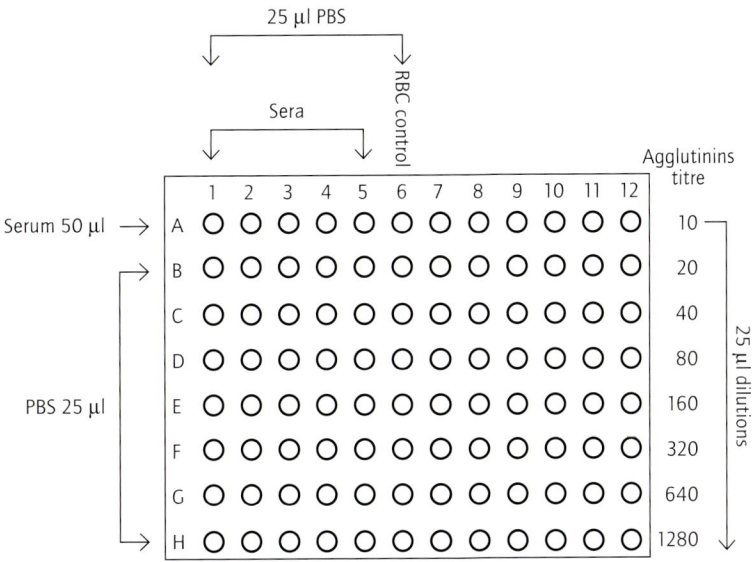

FIGURE 2.E-3
Examples of red blood cell (RBC) agglutination patterns

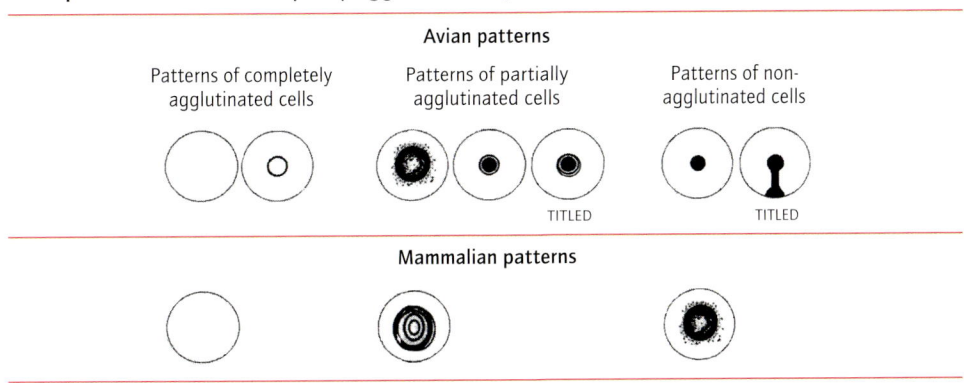

3. Centrifuge at 1200 rpm for 10 minutes.
4. Carefully remove the adsorbed serum without disturbing the packed RBCs.
5. Check for the presence of nonspecific agglutinins in the serum, as described above.
6. Repeat adsorption with RBCs until there is no haemagglutination associated with the serum.

Haemagglutination titration of control antigens and viral isolates

1. Choose the appropriate type of 96-well microtitre plate (**TABLE 2.E-1**) and label 2 plates oriented as shown in **FIGURE 2.E-4**. One plate will be used for the control antigens and a second plate for the viral isolates according to the key shown for **FIGURE 2.E-4**.

FIGURE 2.E-4
Schematic outline of haemagglutination titration of control antigens and viral isolates

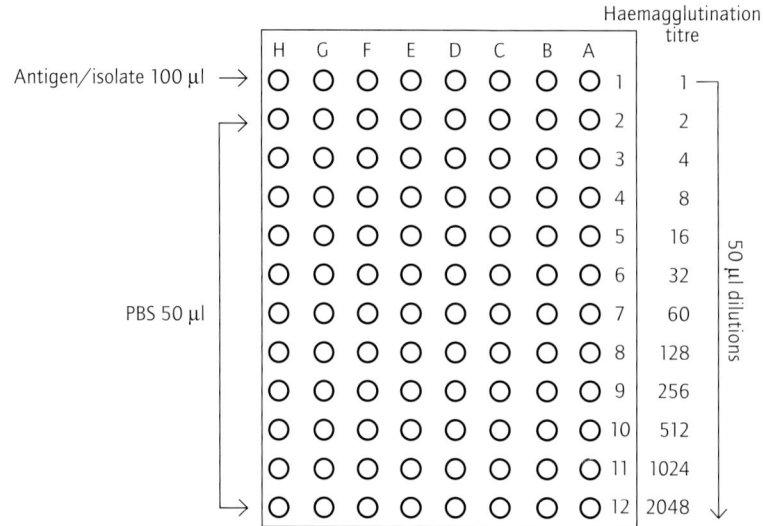

Key to FIGURE 2.E-4

Plate 1: control antigens
A – Influenza A(H1) control antigen
B – Influenza A(H3) control antigen
C – Influenza B control antigen (B/Yamagata/16/88 lineage)
D – Influenza B control antigen (B/Victoria/02/87 lineage)
E – Influenza B ether-treated control antigen (B/Yamagata/16/88)[a]
F – Influenza B ether-treated control antigen (B/Victoria/02/87)[a]
G – Blank
H – RBC control (PBS)

Plate 2: viral isolates
A – Viral isolate 1
B – Viral isolate 2
C – Viral isolate 3
D – Viral isolate 4
E – Viral isolate 5
F – Viral isolate 6
G – Viral isolate 7
H – RBC control (PBS)

[a] Ether-treated control antigens are included for use in serological diagnosis.

2. Add 50 μl PBS (pH 7.2) to wells 2 to 12 of each row (i.e. A2–A12; B2–B12; etc. up to H2–H12).
3. For plate 1, add 100 μl of each control antigen to the first wells of rows A–F (i.e. A1–F1). For plate 2, add 100 μl of each different viral isolate to the first wells of rows A–G (i.e. A1–G1 to allow for the testing of up to 7 different isolates).
4. For both plates, prepare an RBC control in row H (well H1) by adding 50 μl PBS.
5. Make serial 2-fold dilutions by transferring 50 μl from the first to successive wells of each row (i.e. A1 to A2; A2 to A3; etc. up to A11 to A12). Discard the final 50 μl.
6. Add 50 μl of standardized RBCs to each well.
7. Mix using a laboratory shaker for 10 seconds or by manually agitating the plates thoroughly.
8. Cover and incubate the plates at room temperature. Check the RBC control for complete settling of the cells.
9. Record and interpret the results.

Interpretation of results

Complete haemagglutination is considered to have occurred when the RBCs are still in suspension after the RBC control has settled completely. This is recorded as a "+". When a portion of the RBCs are partially agglutinated (or partially settled) a "+/-" is used.

Non-agglutinated chicken or turkey RBCs form a compact button on the bottom of the wells. The absence of haemagglutination can be confirmed by tilting the plates at a 45-degree angle for 20–30 seconds. If the settled RBCs "run" or form a tear-drop at the same rate as the controls then that particular well is considered negative for agglutination. Non-agglutinated guinea-pig or human type O RBCs appear as a halo or circle of settled cells on the bottom of the wells. A "0" is used to record the absence of haemagglutination in all these types of RBC.

The haemagglutination titration **end-point** is defined as the highest dilution of virus that still causes complete haemagglutination. The haemagglutination **titre** is the reciprocal of this dilution. For example, if a virus causes complete haemagglutination up to a 1:256 dilution then the HA titre of the virus stock is 256.

One **unit** of haemagglutination is contained in the end-point dilution of the HA titration. The unit of haemagglutination is an operational unit dependent upon the volumes used for haemagglutination titration. A haemagglutination unit is defined as the amount of antigen (virus) needed to agglutinate an equal volume of a standardized RBC suspension.

Preparation of standardized antigen (control antigens and viral isolates) for the HAI test and back titration

1. Determine the volume of standardized antigen needed for the HAI test. For example, 1 ml of standardized antigen will test 5 sera, each of which is diluted in 8 wells with 25 µl of antigen added to each well (25 x 8 x 5 = 1 ml standardized antigen). Prepare an additional 1 ml for back titration and wastage.
2. Determine the dilution of standardized antigen needed for the test. In the test, 4 haemagglutination units of antigen are added to 2-fold dilutions of sera. Since 25 µl of standardized antigen is added to each well, a dilution that contains 4 haemagglutination units per 25 µl (equivalent to 8 units per 50 µl) is needed. To calculate the antigen dilution needed for the assay, divide the haemagglutination titre (which is based on 50 µl) by 8. For example, a haemagglutination titre of 160 divided by 8 is 20. Mix 1 part of antigen with 19 parts of PBS (pH 7.2) to obtain the desired volume of standardized antigen (e.g. add 0.1 ml of antigen to 1.9 ml of PBS).
3. Prepare the dilution. Keep a record of the dilution prepared using the influenza antigen unit standardization worksheet provided in **ANNEX IV**.
4. Perform a back titration to verify the correct units of haemagglutination by performing a second haemagglutination test, using the standardized antigen dilution preparation. Store the diluted antigen at 4 °C and use within the same day.
5. Record and interpret the results on the sheet provided in **ANNEX IV**.

Standardized antigens must have a haemagglutination titre of 4 haemagglutination units per 25 µl (equivalent to 8 units per 50 µl). This titre will haemagglutinate the first four wells of a row of a back-titration plate. If an antigen does not have a titre of 8 per 50 µl it must be adjusted accordingly by adding more antigen (to increase the number of units) or by diluting (to decrease the number of units). For example, if complete haemagglutination is present in the fifth well, the antigen has a titre of 16 and should be diluted 2-fold. Conversely, if haemagglutination is only present up to the third well, the antigen has a titre of 4 and a volume of antigen equal to that used when the antigen was initially diluted must be added. This will double the concentration of antigen in the test dilution to give a titre of 8 units. Continue adjusting the concentration of antigen until 4 haemagglutination units per 25 μl (8 units per 50 μl) is obtained.

Procedure for identifying viral isolates using HAI testing

1. Choose the appropriate type of 96-well microtitre plate (**TABLE 2.E-1**) and label the plates as shown in **FIGURE 2.E-5**.
2. Two antigens/isolates can be used per plate so that a complete set of sera (usually 5) can be tested. An extra plate is required as a serum control and is set up identically except that PBS is added instead of antigen. Determine the number of plates to be set up bearing in mind that a complete set of RDE-treated reference sera should include:
   — influenza A(H1N1) antiserum;
   — influenza A(H3N2) antiserum;
   — influenza B (B/Yamagata/16/88 lineage) antiserum;
   — influenza B (B/Victoria/02/87 lineage) antiserum; and
   — negative control serum.
3. Add 25 μl PBS to the wells in rows B to H (i.e. B1–B12; C1–C12; etc. up to H1–H12).
4. Using the set of 5 RDE-treated sera (which are already diluted 1:10) add 50 μl of each serum to the first well of the appropriate column (in duplicate). For example, serum 1 should be added to well A1 and well A8; serum 2 to A2 and A9; etc.
5. Add 50 μl PBS to the first wells of columns 6 and 7 (i.e. A6 and A7) for RBC controls.
6. Prepare serial 2-fold dilutions of the treated sera by transferring 25 μl from the first to successive wells of a column (i.e. A1–H1; A2–H2, etc.). Discard the final 25 μl after row H.
7. Add 25 μl standardized control antigen 1 to all wells of a complete set of diluted treated sera (e.g. A1–H5). Continue with the other standardized control antigens and viral isolates. ***Note: the 4 haemagglutination units in these 25 μl volumes are added to the test because the haemagglutination unit calculations are based upon a volume of 50 μl***.
8. Add 25 μl PBS instead of antigen to the serum control plate.
9. Mix the contents of the plates using a laboratory shaker for 10 seconds or by manually agitating the plates thoroughly.
10. Cover the plates and incubate at room temperature for 15 minutes.
11. Add 50 μl of standardized RBCs to all wells. Mix as in step **9**.
12. Cover the plates and allow the RBCs to settle at room temperature for the appropriate time according to the RBCs being used (**TABLE 2.E-1**).
13. Record the HAI titres on the sheet provided in **ANNEX V**.

FIGURE 2.E-5
Schematic outline for identifying viral isolates using HAI testing

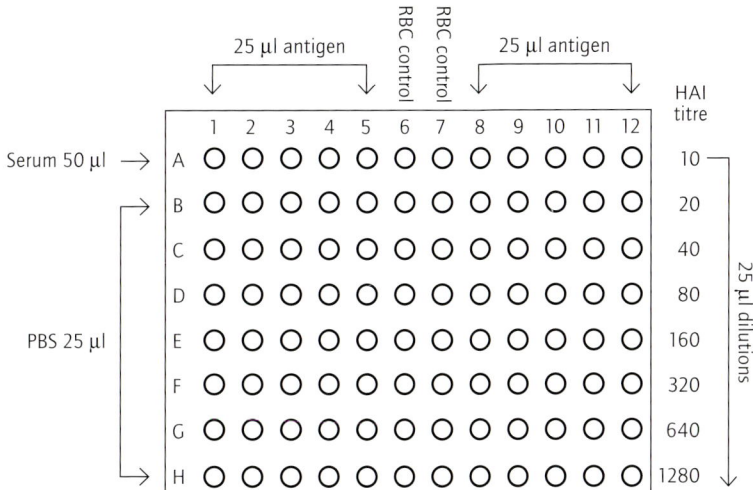

Key to FIGURE 2.E-5
A1 – Influenza A(H1) reference antiserum
A2 – Influenza A(H3) reference antiserum
A3 – Influenza B reference antiserum (B/Yamagata/16/88 lineage)
A4 – Influenza B reference antiserum (B/Victoria/02/87 lineage)
A5 – Negative control serum
A6 – RBC control (PBS)
A7 – RBC control (PBS)
A8 – Influenza A(H1) reference antiserum
A9 – Influenza A(H3) reference antiserum
A10 – Influenza B reference antiserum (B/Yamagata/16/88 lineage)
A11 – Influenza B reference antiserum (B/Victoria/02/87 lineage)
A12 – Negative control serum

Interpretation of results

If an antigen-antibody reaction does occur then haemagglutination of the RBCs will be inhibited. An illustration of the use of such HAI reactions in the identification of viral isolates is shown in **FIGURE 2.E-6**. In this example, viral isolate 1 is identified as influenza A(H3) and viral isolate 2 as influenza A(H1) when compared with the control antigens. An insignificant cross-reaction with influenza A(H3N2) reference antisera and viral isolate 2 is shown in column 9. The RBC controls in columns 6 and 7 are correct.

To identify a viral isolate, the results for each isolate should be compared with those for the antigen controls. A viral isolate is identified as a particular type or subtype if it reacts with one reference antiserum at a 4-fold or greater HAI titre than it reacts with other antisera. The HAI titre is then the reciprocal of the highest dilution of antiserum that completely inhibits haemagglutination.

An example of how to interpret HAI titre results obtained for viral isolates using the WHO Influenza Reagent Kit is shown in **TABLE 2.E-2**. The influenza A identifications are clear: isolate 2 is influenza A(H1) with some cross-reactivity with influenza A(H3N2) antiserum. Isolate 5 is influenza A(H3) with insignificant low-level cross-reactivity with influenza A(H1N1) antiserum. Cross-reactions between influenza B viruses require careful interpretation. Viral isolates that are B/Yamagata/16/88-like will cross-react with refer-

FIGURE 2.E-6
Identification of viral isolates – an illustration of HAI reactions

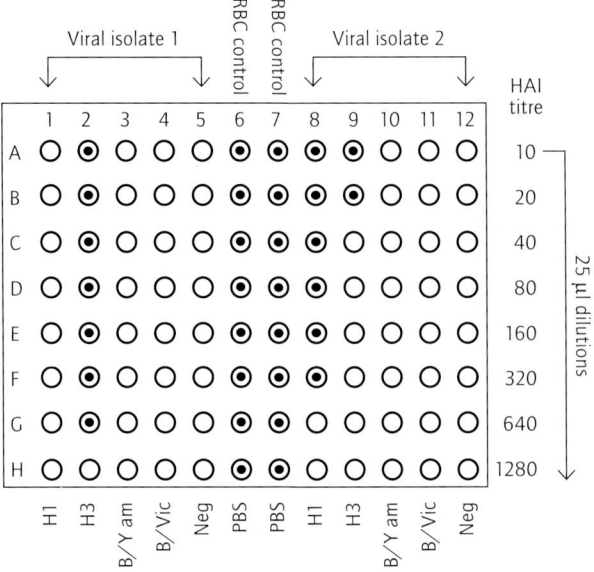

Controls: H1 – A(H1) reference antiserum; **H3** – A(H3) reference antiserum; **B/Yam** – B/Yamagata/16/88 lineage reference antiserum; **B/Vic** – B/Victoria/02/87 lineage reference antiserum; **Neg** – negative control serum; **PBS** – phosphate-buffered saline; **RBC** – red blood cell.

ence antiserum to B/Victoria/02/87 lineage, as can be seen with isolate 3. Even when the cross-reaction with B/Victoria/02/87 lineage antiserum is greater than shown in **TABLE 2.E-2**, the correct interpretation is B/Yamagata/16/88-like. In contrast, B/Victoria/02/87-like viruses are specific and do not cross-react with B/Yamagata/16/88 lineage antiserum, as seen with isolates 1, 4 and 8. This one-way cross-reaction has been verified in numerous tests and has also been confirmed by sequencing.

Limitations of the HAI test and potential problems in its interpretation
Limitations

The evolution of influenza viruses can result in changes in host susceptibility. Historically, embryonated eggs have been the host of choice for influenza virus isolation from clinical specimens. However, difficulties can be encountered when using eggs for the isolation (and passaging) of some strains of influenza viruses. Most laboratories now perform primary virus isolation using MDCK or primary rhesus monkey kidney cell cultures. The observed reduction in the haemagglutination titre of isolates grown in cell culture compared with egg-grown isolates is a limitation of cell culture systems.

Variability between different passage levels of MDCK cells and between batches of primary monkey kidney cells can also affect influenza virus replication. With MDCK cell culture, the passage level range that is optimally sensitive to viral replication must be established by the laboratory and adequate seed stocks of frozen cell suspensions must be kept to re-establish sensitivity as required.

TABLE 2.E-2
Haemagglutination inhibition (HAI) reaction of the WHO Influenza Reagent Kit

	Antigens	HAI titres using reference sera[a]					Interpretation[b]
		A(H1N1)	A(H3N2)	B/Yam	B/Vic	Negative	
Control antigens							
1	A(H1N1)	≥1280	<10	<10	<10	<10	
2	A(H3N2)	<10	≥1280	20	<10	<10	
3	B/Yam	<10	<10	320	40	<10	
4	B/Vic	<10	<10	<10	320	<10	
2002–2003 viral isolates							
5	Viral isolate 1	<10	<10	<10	320	<10	B/Vic/02/87-like
6	Viral isolate 2	≥1280	40	<10	<10	<10	A(H1)
7	Viral isolate 3	<10	<10	160	20	<10	B/Yam/16/88-like
8	Viral isolate 4	<10	<10	<10	320	<10	B/Vic/02/87-like
9	Viral isolate 5	20	≥1280	<10	<10	<10	A(H3)
10	Viral isolate 6	<10	≥1280	20	<10	<10	A(H3)
11	Viral isolate 7	≥1280	<10	<10	<10	<10	A(H1)
12	Viral isolate 8	<10	<10	<10	320	<10	B/Vic/02/87-like
13	Viral isolate 9	<10	640	<10	<10	<10	A(H3)
14	Viral isolate 10	≥1280	20	<10	<10	<10	A(H1)

[a] All reference sera are sheep sera. The negative control is uninfected sheep serum. All sera are treated with RDE from the WHO Influenza Reagent Kit.
[b] If cross-reactivity between different antisera occurs with some viral isolates, identification of these isolates should be based on a 4-fold or greater difference in HAI titre.
B/Yam – influenza B/Yamagata/16/88 lineage.
B/Vic – influenza B/Victoria/02/87 lineage.

There are also differences in the ability of different influenza viruses to agglutinate RBCs. Amino acid changes located in and around the receptor binding pocket of the viral HA molecule sometimes result in a loss of sensitivity to certain RBCs. Turkey RBCs are frequently chosen for HAI testing because the settling time is shorter, inhibition patterns are clearer and the cells are readily available. However, it is known that some strains of influenza viruses during initial and early passage may react poorly to turkey RBCs. Guinea-pig RBCs have consistently been demonstrated to be more sensitive in detecting human influenza viruses and should therefore be used for maximum sensitivity when detecting newly isolated viruses.

Problems of interpretation

Potential causes of problems in interpreting the results of HAI testing include:

- **Nonspecific inhibitors of haemagglutination present in serum** – as outlined above, certain non-antibody molecules present in serum are capable of binding to the viral HA, resulting in nonspecific inhibition and the incorrect interpretation of results. The binding is believed to occur because these serum components contain sialic acid residues that mimic the receptors of RBCs and thus compete with RBC receptors for the viral HA. Three molecular types of inhibitor (designated alpha, beta and gamma) have been described in human or animal sera. These inhibitors exhibit different levels of activity against the HA of different influenza viral strains. To perform a valid HAI test, care must therefore be taken to ensure that the serum does not contain any non-specific inhibitors that react with the virus antigen being tested. Several methods exist for inactivating nonspecific inhibitors in sera of different species. When nonspecific inhibitors create a problem with the interpretation in HAI tests, different treatment methods may need to be considered. The inactivation procedure described previously in this section is specific to the RDE supplied in the WHO Influenza Reagent Kit.

- **Viral isolates that are highly sensitive to the nonspecific inhibitors of haemagglutination present in sera** – the inhibitors are not always completely removed by RDE treatment and their presence can give false positives. Occasionally isolates are seen that are highly sensitive in this respect and these will usually have high HAI titres to more than one antiserum in the test. Such results must therefore be interpreted with care.
- **The presence of nonspecific agglutinins in sera** – if any haemagglutination occurs in the serum controls it is due to nonspecific agglutinins in the sera. Their presence can produce false-negatives. The adsorption of treated sera to remove such nonspecific agglutinins is also outlined above.

In order to address such limitations and problems in interpretation, and to ensure optimal HAI test performance when identifying viral isolates or diagnosing infections serologically, it is essential that test procedures be followed exactly. The following points should be noted:

- Standardized antigen dilutions must contain 4 haemagglutination units per 25 µl. The antigen dilutions must be prepared and back titrated each test day.
- Incubation times must be strictly observed. Plates must be read promptly when the RBC control has completely settled. Elution of RBCs from the antigen can occur with some virus strains. When this happens, the plates may be read earlier or placed at 4 °C.
- RBC suspensions must be standardized consistently.
- Test reagents must be handled and stored in the prescribed manner. To minimize freeze-thawing and to avoid bacterial contamination, dispense reagents in small volumes using sterile techniques.
- Lyophilized reagents should be reconstituted to the volume described and stored according to instructions.
- Depending on the choice of RBCs, appropriate microtitre plates (U-shaped or V-shaped) must be used.
- Avoid bacterial contamination by using sterile techniques and by dispensing reagents in usable aliquots. Agglutinins of non-influenza viral origin in contaminated specimens may interfere the test and its interpretation.

It is also essential to include appropriate controls as part of ensuring the quality of HAI testing when identifying viral isolates. The following points should be noted:

- RBC controls allow for adjustments in incubation times. There should be an RBC control on each plate if possible.

- Each viral isolate and the control antigens must be tested with a negative serum control. The negative serum control will allow for the identification of anti-host component antibodies. When such antibodies occur (as has been observed with influenza B viruses isolated in MDCK cells) the sera may be adsorbed with uninfected host cells to remove the anti-host component antibodies.
- Serum controls are required for all sera in order to detect nonspecific agglutinins, which must be removed.
- Viral isolates and control antigens must be tested with all antisera provided in the WHO Influenza Reagent Kit. The reactions of the control antigens will permit the accurate identification of the viral isolate.
- Appropriate record sheets (as provided in **ANNEX IV** and **ANNEX V**) should be kept of each test performed in order to monitor reproducibility.

2.F
Serological diagnosis of influenza by haemagglutination inhibition testing

Diagnosing influenza by virus isolation definitively identifies the infecting strain and is usually more rapid than serological diagnosis. However, serological diagnosis is an important approach when clinical specimens are unobtainable or when a laboratory does not have the resources required for virus isolation. Many laboratories rely on serology for diagnosing recent individual infections. Such individual diagnosis must be based on acute-phase and convalescent-phase sera collected two to three weeks apart. The antibody response will usually be reflected by a rise in titre to one viral type or subtype. Demonstration of an acute influenza infection using serology requires a significant increase in antibody titres (i.e. 4-fold or greater) between acute-phase and convalescent-phase serum samples. The demonstration of such a significant increase may establish the diagnosis of a recent infection even when attempts to detect the virus are negative. Serological methods such as the HAI test are also essential for epidemiological and immunological studies; for evaluation of the antibody response following vaccination; and in certain situations where identification of the virus is not otherwise feasible (e.g. after viral shedding has stopped).

Since most human sera contain antibodies to influenza viruses, diagnosis of individual cases using a single convalescent-phase serum is unreliable and should generally not be attempted. Although a single serum sample is unreliable for individual diagnosis, single serum samples can be used for presumptive diagnosis during an outbreak situation. If a statistically significant number of sera are collected from individuals in the acute phase of illness and an equal number are collected from individuals (matched according to age) in the convalescent phase of illness, then the sera can be tested simultaneously for antibodies. Based on geometric mean titres, a significant statistical difference between the two groups must be demonstrated before the outbreak can be confirmed to be influenza.

Alternatively, single serum samples can be collected from cases bled several weeks after symptom onset and then paired with those from age-matched and apparently healthy control individuals during the outbreak or from historical bleeds before the outbreak. In this approach, analysis is more difficult since apparently healthy people or historical controls may have antibody titres sufficiently high enough to obscure the current antibodies. This could happen for various reasons, such as an apparently healthy person having an asymptomatic infection or, in the case of historical controls, there may have been an undocumented influenza virus circulating in the population.

Although other diagnostic tests such as complement fixation and enzyme immunoassay can be used for serological diagnosis, the HAI test is preferred. Reagents for serological diagnosis using the HAI test are provided in the WHO Influenza Reagent Kit (see **SECTION 2.E**). Influenza A antigens contained in the kit are suitable for the serological diagnosis of influenza A(H1) or A(H3) infections. Due to the decreased sensitivity to antibody rises of influenza B whole viral antigens, ether-treated antigens are required for use in the serological diagnosis of influenza B infections – these are also provided in the kit.

Procedures for serological diagnosis using the HAI test

Carry out the following procedures (see **SECTION 2.E** for detailed protocols and materials required):

- Treatment of test and reference sera with RDE to inactivate nonspecific inhibitors of haemagglutination. Always include:
  — influenza A(H1N1) antiserum;
  — influenza A(H3N2) antiserum;
  — influenza B (B/Yamagata/16/88 lineage) antiserum;
  — influenza B (B/Victoria/02/87 lineage) antiserum; and
  — negative control serum.
- Adsorption of treated test and reference sera to remove nonspecific agglutinins.
- Standardization of RBCs.
- Haemagglutination titration of control antigens. The 4 control antigens in the WHO kit are:
  — influenza A(H1N1);
  — influenza A(H3N2);
  — ether-treated influenza B/Yamagata/16/88 lineage; and
  — ether-treated influenza B/Victoria/02/87 lineage.
- Preparation of standardized control antigens for the HAI test and back titration. Each control antigen must be standardized to contain 4 haemagglutination units per 25 µl (8 units per 50 µl).

HAI test for serological diagnosis

1. Choose the appropriate type of 96-well microtitre plate and label the plates as shown in **FIGURE 2.F-1**. One set of reference sera will be needed for each antigen to be tested, as well as a set for a serum control (see step **6**). Thus if the 4 control antigens from the WHO kit are being used, 5 sets of sera will be needed.
2. Add 25 µl PBS (pH 7.2) to the wells in **rows** B to H (B1–B12; C1–C12, etc. up to H1–H12).
3. Add 50 µl of each treated serum (diluted 1:10) to the appropriate well in row A (A1–A12).
4. Prepare serial 2-fold dilutions of the treated sera by transferring 25 µl from the first to successive wells of each **column** (i.e. A1–H1; A2–H2, etc.). Discard the final 25 µl after row H.
5. Add 25 µl standardized antigen to all wells (A1–H12) of plates containing the sets of treated sera.
6. Add 25 µl PBS instead of antigen to all wells (A1–H12) of the plate containing the set of treated sera to be used as serum controls.
7. Mix the contents of the plates using a laboratory shaker for 10 seconds or by manually agitating the plates thoroughly.
8. Cover the plates and incubate at room temperature for 15 minutes.
9. Add 50 µl standardized RBCs to all wells. Mix as in step 7.

FIGURE 2.F-1
Schematic outline of serological diagnosis by HAI

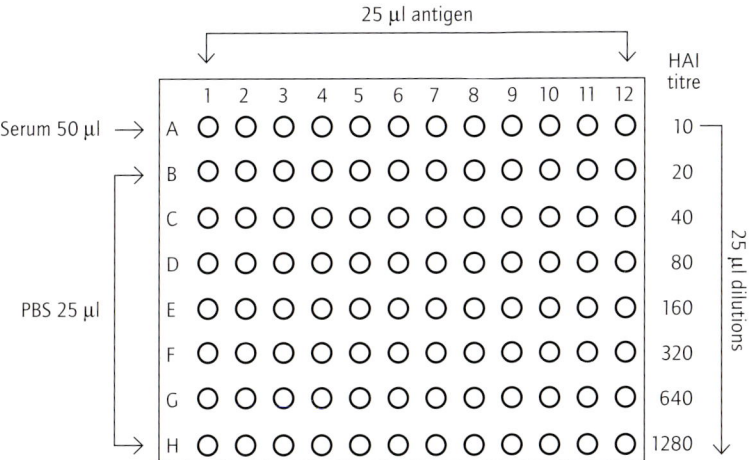

Key to FIGURE 2.F-1
1 – Test serum 1 (S1) – refers to acute-phase (or first) serum
2 – Test serum 1 (S2) – refers to convalescent-phase (or second) serum
3 – Test serum 2 (S1)
4 – Test serum 2 (S2)
5 – Test serum 3 (S1)
6 – Test serum 3 (S2)
7 – Influenza A(H1N1) reference antiserum
8 – Influenza A(H3N2) reference antiserum
9 – Influenza B (B/Yamagata/16/88 lineage) reference antiserum
10 – Influenza B (B/Victoria/02/87 lineage) reference antiserum
11 – Negative control serum
12 – Red blood cell (RBC) control (PBS)

10. Cover the plates and allow the RBCs to settle at room temperature for the appropriate time according to the RBCs being used.
11. Record the HAI titres (see **ANNEX VI**) and interpret the results.

Interpretation of results

Haemagglutination and its inhibition are read as described in **SECTION 2.E**. The control antigens and corresponding reference antisera should give consistent results when compared with previous tests. A 4-fold increase in titre between the acute-phase (S1) and convalescent-phase (S2) serum is considered diagnostically positive for that particular influenza type or subtype. An illustration of HAI reactions for serological diagnosis is shown in **FIGURE 2.F-2** along with the interpretation of the results.

Interpretation of results
- **Test serum 1** – a 2-fold rise in titre is interpreted as evidence of pre-existing antibodies to A(H3) probably not related to a recent infection.
- **Test serum 2** – a greater than 4-fold rise in titre is interpreted as diagnostically significant and indicative of a recent infection by an influenza A(H3) virus.
- **Test serum 3** – a 4-fold rise is indicative of a recent infection by an influenza A(H3) virus.

FIGURE 2.F-2
Serological diagnosis – illustration of HAI reactions using influenza A(H3) control antigen

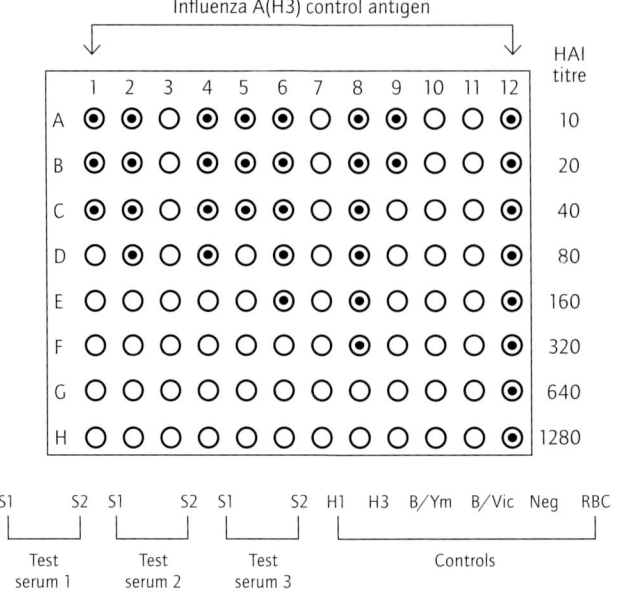

Key to FIGURE 2.F-2
S1 – acute-phase (or first) serum
S2 – convalescent-phase (or second) serum
H1 – A(H1N1) reference antiserum
H3 – A(H3N2) reference antiserum
B/Yam – B/Yamagata/16/88 lineage reference antiserum
B/Vic – B/Victoria/02/87 lineage reference antiserum
Neg – negative control antiserum
RBC – red blood cell

2.G Serological diagnosis of influenza by microneutralization assay

Serological methods rarely yield an early diagnosis of acute influenza virus infection. However, the demonstration of a significant increase in antibody titres (greater than or equal to 4-fold) between acute-phase and convalescent-phase sera may establish the diagnosis of a recent influenza infection even when attempts to detect the virus are negative. Apart from their retrospective diagnostic value, serological methods such as virus neutralization and haemagglutination inhibition are the fundamental tools in epidemiological and immunological studies, as well as in the evaluation of vaccine immunogenicity.

The microneutralization assay is a highly sensitive and specific assay for detecting virus-specific neutralizing antibodies to influenza viruses in human and animal sera, potentially including the detection of human antibodies to avian subtypes. Virus neutralization gives the most precise answer to the question of whether or not an individual has antibodies that can neutralize the infectivity of a given virus strain. The assay has several additional advantages in detecting antibodies to influenza virus. First, it primarily detects antibodies to the influenza viral HA protein and thus can identify functional strain-specific antibodies in human and animal sera. Second, since infectious virus is used, the assay can be carried out quickly once the emergence of a novel virus is recognized. Although conventional neutralization tests for influenza viruses (based on the inhibition of cytopathogenic effect formation in MDCK cell culture) are laborious and rather slow, a microneutralization assay using microtitre plates in combination with an ELISA to detect virus-infected cells can yield results within two days.

On day 1, the following two-step procedure is performed:

1. a virus-antibody reaction step, in which the virus is mixed with dilutions of serum and time allowed for any antibodies to react; and
2. an inoculation step, in which the mixture is inoculated into the appropriate host system – MDCK cells in the case of the following assay.

On day 2, an ELISA is then performed to detect virus-infected cells. The absence of infectivity constitutes a positive neutralization reaction and indicates the presence of virus-specific antibodies in the serum sample. In cases of influenza-like illness, paired acute and convalescent serum samples are preferred. An acute sample should be collected within seven days of symptom onset and the convalescent sample collected at least 14 days after the acute sample, and ideally within 1–2 months of the onset of illness. A 4-fold or great rise in antibody titre demonstrates a seroconversion and is considered to be diagnostic. With single-serum samples, care must be taken in interpreting low titres such as 20 and 40. Generally, knowledge of the antibody titres in an age-matched control population is needed to determine the minimum titre that is indicative of a specific antibody response to the virus used in the assay.

The influenza virus microneutralization assay presented below is based on the assumption that serum-neutralizing antibodies to influenza viral HA will inhibit the infection of MDCK cells with virus. Serially diluted sera should be pre-incubated with a standardized amount of virus before the addition of MDCK cells. After overnight incubation, the cells are fixed and the presence of influenza A virus nucleoprotein (NP) protein in infected cells is detected by ELISA. The microneutralization protocol is therefore divided into three parts:

Part I: Determination of the tissue culture infectious dose (TCID).
Part II: Virus microneutralization assay.
Part III: ELISA.

An overview of the microneutralization assay is shown in FIGURE 2-G-1 and an assay process sheet is provided in ANNEX VII.

FIGURE 2.G-1
Overview of the microneutralization assay

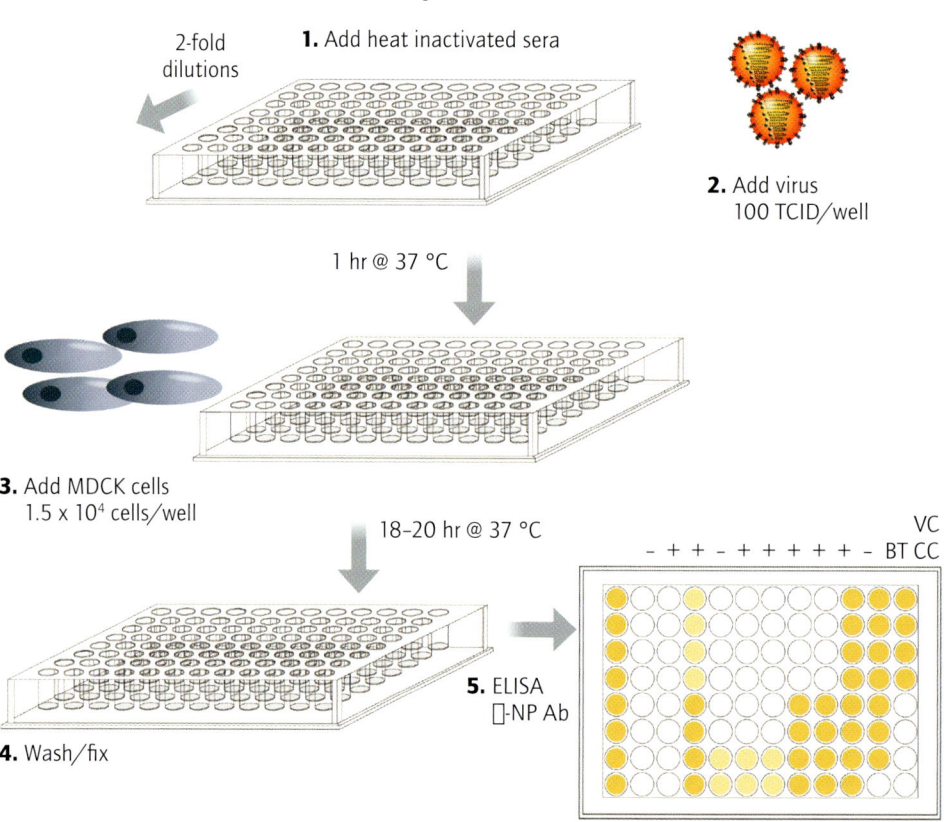

Materials required

Equipment

Water-bath (37 °C)	Water-bath (56 °C)
Automatic ELISA reader with 490 nm filter	Incubator (humidified, 37 °C; 5% CO2)
Automatic plate washer (not essential but would be optimal)	Microscope (inverted or standard)
Centrifuge (low speed; benchtop; preferably with refrigeration) **Sorvall – cat. no. 75006434**	

Supplies

Cell culture flasks (162 cm^2, sterile, vented) **Corning Life Sciences – cat. no. 3151**	Cryovials (2 ml, sterile) **Wheaton Science – cat. no. 985731**
96-well microtitre plates (flat-bottom, Immulon-2HB plates) **Thermo – cat. no. 3455**	Pipettes (assorted sizes, sterile)
Haemacytometer (double rule "bright line") **Reichert – cat. no. 1490**	Haemacytometer coverslips **Reichert – cat. no. 1492**
Cell counter (2-unit counter) **Fisher Scientific – cat. no. 02-670-12**	Tips for Pipetman (sterile) **Rainin – cat. no. RT-20**
Multichannel pipetter **Rainin – cat. no. L12-200**	Tips for multichannel pipetter **Rainin – cat. no. RT-L200F**
Pipetman (1–200 µl) **Rainin – cat. no. P-200**	

Cells, media and buffers

MDCK cell culture monolayer – low passage (<25–30 passages) at low crowding (70–95% confluence)	MDCK sterile cell culture maintenance medium (see below)
D-MEM high glucose (1x) liquid, with L-glutamine and without sodium pyruvate **Invitrogen – cat. no. 11965-092**	HEPES buffer (1 M stock solution) **Invitrogen – cat. no. 15630-080**
Antibody diluents (see below)	Wash buffer (see below)
0.01 M PBS (pH 7.2) **Invitrogen – cat. no. 20012-043**	Citrate buffer capsules (optional) **Sigma – cat. no. P4922**
Water (distilled and deionized)	

Reagents

Penicillin-streptomycin (stock solution contains 10 000 U/ml penicillin; and 10 000 µg/ml streptomycin sulfate) **Invitrogen – cat. no. 15140-122**	Fetal bovine serum (FBS) **Hyclone – cat. no. SH30070.03**
200 mM L-glutamine **Invitrogen – cat. no. 25030-081**	Bovine albumin fraction V (prepared as a 10% solution in water) **Roche – cat. no. 03117332001**
Trypsin-EDTA (0.05% trypsin; 0.53 mM EDTA · 4Na) **Invitrogen – cat. no. 25300-054**	Non-fat dry milk **Fisher Scientific – cat. no. 15260-037**
Tween 20 **Sigma – cat. no. P1379**	Ethanol (70%) **Fisher Scientific – cat. no. S71822**
Trypsin – TPCK-treated (type XIII from bovine pancreas) **Sigma – cat. no. T1426**	Trypan blue stain (0.4%) **Invitrogen – cat. no. 15250-061**
o-phenylenediamine dihydrochloride (OPD) **Sigma – cat. no. P8287**	Acetone **Fisher Scientific – cat. no. A18-500**
Virus diluent (see below)	Fixative (see below)
Stop solution (see below)	

Antibodies

Anti-influenza A NP mouse monoclonal antibody **United States Centers for Disease Control and Prevention – cat. no. VS2208**	Goat anti-mouse IgG conjugated to horseradish peroxidase (HRP), lyophilized **Kirkegaard and Perry Laboratories Inc. – cat. no. 074-1802**

Preparation of media and solutions

MDCK sterile cell culture maintenance medium

a. To 500 ml D-MEM, add 5.5 ml 100x antibiotics.
b. Add 5.5 ml 200 mM L-glutamine.
c. Add 50 ml FBS that has been heat-inactivated at 56 °C for 30 minutes.

Virus diluent (make fresh)

a. To 500 ml D-MEM, add 58 ml of bovine albumin fraction V (10%).
b. Add 6 ml 100x antibiotics.
c. Add 12.5 ml of 1 M HEPES.

Fixative (make fresh and chill to -20 °C before use)

a. To 100 ml 0.01 M PBS (pH 7.2) add 400 ml acetone.
b. Store at -20 °C until just before use.

PBS (0.01 M, pH 7.2)

a. In 800 ml of distilled deionized water, dissolve:
- 8.0 g sodium chloride (NaCl);
- 0.20 g potassium chloride (KCl);

— 1.15 g dibasic anhydrous sodium phosphate (Na_2HPO_4); and
— 0.21 g monobasic anhydrous potassium phosphate (KH_2PO_4).
b. Adjust pH to 7.2 with HCl and bring volume up to 1 litre with distilled deionized water.
c. Sterilize by autoclaving.

Wash buffer

To 1 litre PBS add 3 ml Tween 20 using a 3 ml or 5 ml syringe with an attached wide-bore blunt-end needle. Wipe the outside of the needle, submerge the tip of the needle, and dispense directly into the PBS while it is vigorously being stirred with a stir bar. Prepare fresh each day.

Antibody diluent

To 1 litre of wash buffer add 50 g non-fat dry milk. Mix using a stir bar for at least 30 minutes before use.

Substrate

a. Prepare a citrate buffer by adding 1 citrate buffer capsule to 100 ml of distilled water.
b. Alternatively, prepare a citrate buffer by adding 29.41 g trisodium citric acid dihydrate (formula weight = 294.10) to 1 litre of distilled water (final concentration = 0.1 M). Adjust pH to 5.0 with HCl. Add 10 µl 30% hydrogen peroxide (0.015% H_2O_2) to each 20 ml of substrate ***just before use***.
c. To 20 ml of either of the above citrate buffers, add 1 OPD tablet (10 mg) ***just before use***.

Stop solution

To 972 ml of distilled water, add 28 ml of stock sulphuric acid (95–98%).

Dye (for determination of cell viability)

Use 0.4% trypan blue stain.

Preparation of antibodies
Primary antibodies

Anti-influenza A NP mouse monoclonal antibody – dilute 1:1000 (or at an optimal concentration determined through testing by the user) in antibody diluent.

Secondary antibody

Goat anti-mouse IgG conjugated to HRP – dilute 1:2000 (or at an optimal concentration determined through testing by the user) in antibody diluent.

Preparation of negative and positive serum controls

If control sera are to be tested repeatedly, it is better to make several aliquots and store them at -20 °C to -70 °C. Both animal and human negative and positive serum controls should be included for each virus used in the assay. Sera should not be repeatedly freeze–

thawed. Human sera need to be heat inactivated at 56 °C for 30 minutes and animal sera require treatment with receptor destroying enzyme (RDE) before use.

Negative (normal) serum control

This is included to determine whether the virus is nonspecifically inactivated by serum components. The negative serum control must be used at the same dilutions as the matching viral antiserum.

- For animal sera, wherever possible use normal serum from the same animal species that is being tested. The best results will be obtained if animal control sera are treated with RDE before use in the assay.
- For human sera, use age-matched normal serum from a population not exposed to the particular virus subtype in question. Human sera must be inactivated at 56 °C for 30 minutes before use in the assay.

Positive (infected or immunized) serum controls

Include antisera to known viruses as positive controls.

- For animal sera, use sera raised in infected ferrets or other immunized animals (sheep, goat, rabbit or mouse). The best results will be obtained if animal control sera are treated with RDE before use in the assay.
- For human sera, optimal positive controls would be acute-phase and convalescent-phase serum samples. Human sera must be inactivated at 56 °C for 30 minutes before use in the assay.

Preparation of virus and cell controls

Viruses in allantoic fluid need to be stored at -70 °C. Determine the virus working dilution before use. Never use any freeze–thawed virus other than the initial freeze–thawed aliquot required to prepare the assay. Include a virus back titration, virus controls (VCs) and cell controls (CCs) with each assay as follows.

Virus titration check (back titration)

1. Add 50 µl of virus diluent to each of the wells A11–H11.
2. Add 50 µl of the working dilution of virus, containing 100x TCID, to well A11. Titrate in 2-fold serial dilutions down the plate (i.e. the 8 wells A11– H11) discarding the last 50 µl from H11. To avoid virus carry-over, change pipette tips between each well.
3. Add an additional 50 µl of virus diluent to the virus titration wells (A11–H11).
4. Incubate for 1 hour at 37 °C in 5% CO_2.
5. Add 100 µl MDCK cells (1.5 x 10^4/well) and then incubate for 18–20 hours (at 37 °C in 5% CO_2) with the rest of the assay.

Positive virus controls (VCs) and negative cell controls (CCs)

Set up 4 wells as positive VCs (50 µl medium + 50 µl working dilution of virus + 100 µl MDCK cells) and 4 wells as negative CCs (100 µl virus diluent + 100 µl MDCK cells) and assay in parallel with the neutralization test. These controls must be included on each plate for analysis of the data on that plate.

Part I: Virus titration and determination of tissue culture infectious dose (TCID) for microneutralization assay

Generation of stock virus

Grow virus to a high titre in the allantoic cavity of 10-day-old embryonated hens' eggs (see **SECTION 2.D** for more details on the growing of viruses in eggs). Alternatively, virus can be grown in MDCK cells (see **SECTION 2.C**). Several different dilutions of virus should be inoculated to determine the maximum HA titre.

Aliquot virus immediately in multiple ampoules (of approximately 1 ml) and freeze at -70 °C. Viruses should never be thawed and refrozen.

Virus titration

1. For optimal infectivity, thaw an ampoule of virus just prior to use.
2. Perform titration of virus in quadruplicate.
3. Test at four starting dilutions (10^{-2}, 10^{-3}, 10^{-4} and 10^{-5}) of virus in virus diluent (e.g. 100 µl virus + 9.9 ml virus diluent for the 10^{-2} dilution).
4. Add 100 µl virus diluent with or without TPCK-trypsin[1] (1–2 µg/ml) to all wells, except column 1 of a 96-well microtitre plate.
5. Add 146 µl of virus of 1:100 virus starting dilution to the first wells in column 1 (A1–H1). Perform ½ $\log_{10}$ dilutions of the virus.
6. Transfer 46 µl serially from column 1 (i.e. A1 to A2; A2 to A3; etc. up until A11). Change pipette tips between each well. Discard the 46 µl after the last dilution in column 11. Dilutions will then be 10^{-2}, $10^{-2.5}$, 10^{-3} and so on to 10^{-7}.
7. In a similar way, serially dilute the other virus starting dilutions.
8. Column 12 contains virus diluents only and is the cell control (CC).
9. Place plate(s) in a 37 °C 5% CO_2 incubator for 1 hour. This replicates the conditions of the microneutralization assay.

Preparation of MDCK cells

Note: all cell culture passage work must be performed in a class-II biosafety cabinet to prevent the contamination of cells. In addition, for safety reasons, seasonal and low pathogenic avian viruses, and human serum samples, should be handled in a class-II biosafety cabinet, while highly pathogenic avian influenza microneutralization assays should additionally be performed only in BSL-3+ laboratories.

1. Check the MDCK cell monolayer (which should be 70–95% confluent; see **FIGURE 2.G-2**). Do not allow the cells to overgrow. Typically, a confluent 162 cm^2 flask (approximately 2 x 10^7 cells/flask) should yield enough cells to seed 4–6 96-well microtitre plates. Split the confluent monolayer 1:10 two days before use for optimum yield and growth.
   Note: cells must be in log-phase growth for maximum virus sensitivity.
2. Remove and discard the culture medium from cell monolayer.
3. Gently rinse the cell monolayer with 5 ml trypsin-EDTA and remove with a pipette.
4. Add 5 ml trypsin-EDTA to cover the monolayer.
5. Lie the flask flat and incubate at 37 °C until the monolayer detaches (approximately 3–10 minutes).

---

[1] When determining the TCID of new test viruses, it is best to perform the titration with and without trypsin to determine the optimal conditions for each virus.

FIGURE 2.G-2
Madin-Darby canine kidney cell monolayer confluencies

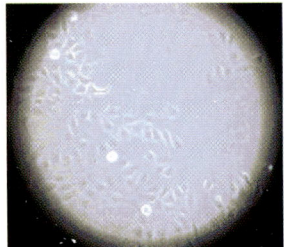 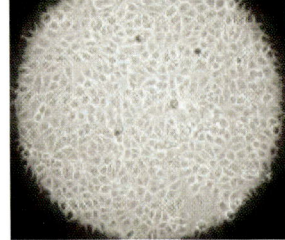 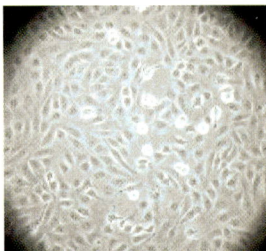

Undergrown cells　　　　　　　　Crowded square cells　　　　　　　Good concentration for use

6. Check flask for dislodgement of the cell monolayer. As soon as most of the monolayer has been dislodged from the bottom of the flask, the remaining cells can be dislodged by gently tapping the sides of the flask.
7. Add 15 ml MDCK sterile cell culture maintenance medium to each flask.
8. Label and fill new 162 cm^2 cell culture flasks with 50 ml MDCK medium.
9. Depending upon when the cells are to be used in the microneutralization assay, cells should be diluted as shown in **TABLE 2.G-1** in the 50 ml MDCK medium in the new 162 cm^2 cell culture flasks. ***Note: the dilutions are based upon optimal growth conditions though some variations may exist***.

TABLE 2.G-1
Dilutions of cell suspensions for passage in 162 cm^2 flasks

Dilution	Volume of cells to add to new flask	When confluent
1:5 (4 ml of the 20 ml)	4 ml	Approximately 1 day
1:10 (2 ml of the 20 ml)	2 ml	Approximately 2 days
1:20 (1 ml of the 20 ml)	1 ml	Approximately 3 days

Preparation of MDCK cells for use in microneutralization assay

1. When ready to perform the assay, wash 70–95% confluent cells with PBS to remove FBS.
2. Add 7 ml trypsin-EDTA to cover the cell monolayer.
3. Lie flask flat and incubate at 37 °C until monolayer detaches (approximately 8–10 minutes).
4. Add 7 ml of virus diluent to each flask.
5. Wash cells twice with virus diluent to remove FBS.
   — gently mix to resuspend and break up clumps of cells;
   — fill tube to 50 ml with virus diluent;
   — pellet cells by centrifugation at 485x g for 5 minutes;
   — decant supernatant; and
   — perform one repeat of the previous 4 steps.
6. Resuspend cells in virus diluent (10 ml per trypsinized flask) and count cells with a

haemacytometer as described below in **Part III, Determination of cell count and viability**.

7. Adjust cell concentration to 1.5×10^5 cells/ml with virus diluent.
8. Add 100 µl diluted cells to each well of the microtitre plate.
9. Incubate cells for 18–20 hours at 37 °C in 5% CO_2.

Determination of cell count and maintenance of MDCK cells

Although estimates can be made of the stage of growth of a cell culture based on its appearance under the microscope, proper quantitative experiments, especially the microneutralization assay, are difficult to assess unless the cells are counted. One of the most critical aspects of the assay is the target cell. Along with the virus infectious dose, the condition and preparation of MDCK cells are the most common causes of assay failure. Optimal growth conditions and appropriate cell concentrations are imperative if the assay is to function properly.

The concentration of cells can be determined by dislodging the adherent cells from the cell culture flask, obtaining a cell suspension, adding an appropriate dye (e.g. trypan blue stain) to distinguish viable from nonviable cells and counting the viable cells on a haemacytometer. The cell number within a defined area of known depth is counted and the concentration is derived from the count.

Fixation of cells

1. Remove medium from microtitre plate.
2. Wash each well with 200 µl PBS.
3. Remove PBS (do not allow wells to dry out) and add 100 µl/well of **cold** fixative.
4. Cover with lid and incubate at room temperature for 10–12 minutes.
5. Remove fixative and let the plate air dry.

Determination of TCID for microneutralization assay

1. Perform ELISA (see protocol below).
2. Calculate the mean absorbance (OD_{490}) of the CCs.
3. Any test well with an OD_{490} greater than twice the OD490 of the CC wells is scored positive for virus growth.
4. Once all test wells have been scored positive or negative for virus growth, the TCID of the virus can be calculated as shown in **TABLE 2.G-2** by the Reed-Muench method (Reed & Muench, 1938).

Calculation

1. Record the number of positive values observed in column (**1**) and negative values in column (**2**) wells of the microtitre plates at each dilution.
2. Calculate the cumulative numbers of positive values in column (**3**) of **TABLE 2.G-2** and negative values in column (**4**) of **TABLE 2.G-2**:
   — column (**3**) – obtained by adding the numbers in column (**1**) starting at the **bottom**.
   — column (**4**) – obtained by adding the numbers in column (**2**) starting at the **top**.
3. Calculate the ratios at each dilution in column (**5**) by dividing the number of positives in column (**3**) by the number of positives plus negatives in columns (**3**) + (**4**).

TABLE 2.G-2
Calculation of tissue culture infectious dose by the Reed-Muench method

Dilution	Observed value (optical density)		Cumulative value			
	(1) No. positive	(2) No. negative	(3) No. positive	(4) No. negative	(5) Ratio	(6) Positive (%)
10^{-4}	8	0	16	0	16/16	100
$10^{-4.5}$	7	1	8	1	8/9	89
10^{-5}	1	7	1	8	1/9	11
$10^{-5.5}$	0	8	0	16	0/16	0

4. Calculate the percentage of positive wells in column (**6**) by converting each of the ratios in column (**5**) to percentages.
5. Calculate the proportional distance between the dilution showing >50% positives in column (**6**) and the dilution showing <50% positives in column (**6**) as follows:

$$\frac{\% \text{ positive value above } 50\% - 50 \times 0.5 \ (\textbf{\textit{correction factor}})}{\% \text{ positive value above } 50\% - \% \text{ positive value below } 50\%}$$

$$= \frac{89 - 50 \times 0.5}{89 - 11} = 0.5 \times 0.5 = 0.25$$

6. The virus working dilution is 200 times the $\log_{10}$ virus dilution at the cut-off point determined by the Reed-Muench method. 200x times the virus dilution at the cut-off point yields a virus working dilution that contains 100x TCID in 50 µl.
7. Calculate the microneutralization TCID by adding the proportional distance to the dilution showing >50% positive. In the above example, add 0.25 to 4.5 to obtain $10^{-4.75}$. The virus working dilution that is 200x the cut-off dilution is $10^{-4.75} \times 200 = 10^{-4.75} + 10^{2.30} = 10^{-2.45} = 1/10^{2.45} = 1:282$. This dilution will give 100x TCID per 50 µl.

If other dilution series are used, other **correction factors** must be used. For example, in this case, the correction factor for a 2-fold dilution series would be 0.3; for a ½ $\log_{10}$ dilution series it would be 0.5; for a 5-fold dilution series it would be 0.7; and for a 10-fold dilution series it would be 1.0 (**TABLE 2.G-3**).

TABLE 2.G-3
Dilution series and correction factors

Dilution series	Correction factor	Example of dilutions
$\log_2$ (2-fold dilutions)	0.3	$2^{-1}, 2^{-2}, 2^{-3}, 2^{-4}$, etc.
½ log10 (½ log dilutions)	0.5	$10^{-2}, 10^{-2.5}, 10^{-3}, 10^{-3.5}$, etc.
$\log_5$ (5-fold dilutions)	0.7	$5^{-1}, 5^{-2}, 5^{-3}, 5^{-4}$, etc.
$\log_{10}$ (10-fold dilutions)	1.0	$10^{-1}, 10^{-2}, 10^{-3}, 10^{-4}$, etc.

Part II: Virus microneutralization assay
Preparation of test antisera

For each virus to be tested once, 10 µl of sera are needed. Sera should be tested in duplicate when possible. A total of 11 sera can be tested on each microtitre plate set up as shown in **FIGURE 2.G-3**. *Note: if assaying for two virus strains, prepare two separate plates*.

1. Heat inactivate sera for 30 minutes at 56 °C.
2. Add 50 µl diluent to each well.
3. Add an additional 40 µl diluent to row A (i.e. wells A1–A11).
4. Add 10 µl heat-inactivated serum per well in row A (e.g. serum 1 in A1; serum 2 in A2, etc.). Do not add serum to well A12.
5. Perform 2-fold serial dilutions by transferring 50 µl progressively from row to row (i.e. A1 to B1; B1 to C1; etc. up to G1 to H1).
6. Discard the final 50 µl after row H.

FIGURE 2.G-3
Virus microneutralization assay

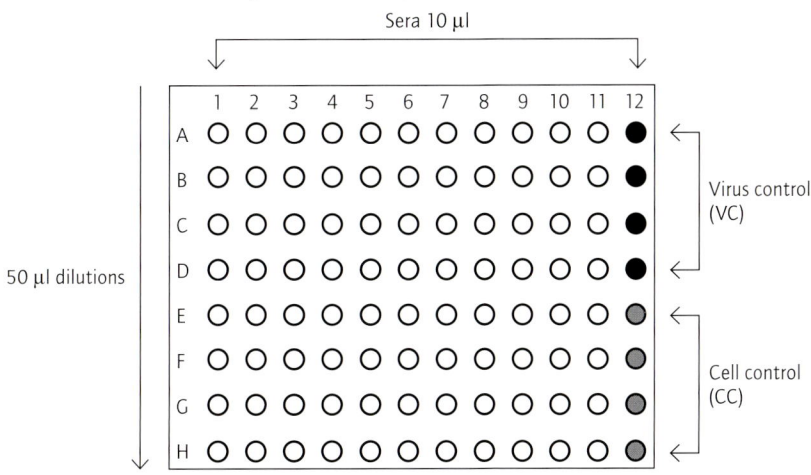

Addition of virus

1. Dilute the virus suspension in virus diluent (± TPCK-trypsin[1]) so that 50 µl contains 100x TCID. Approximately 5 ml/plate is needed. Initial virus titration will determine if the addition of TPCK-trypsin to the diluent is optimal for virus infection of MDCK cells.
2. Add 50 µl diluted virus to all wells (except CC wells E12, F12, G12 and H12).
3. Add 50 µl virus diluent to CC wells.
4. Set up back titration – start with the virus working dilution, 100x TCID in 50 µl, and prepare an additional serial 2-fold dilution with diluent. After dilution, add 50 µl of diluent to each well for a final volume of 100 µl.
5. Incubate the virus-serum mixtures and the virus back titration for 1 hour at 37 °C in 5% CO_2.

---

[1] When determining the TCID of new test viruses, it is best to perform the titration with and without trypsin to determine the optimal conditions for each virus.

Addition of MDCK cells

1. Prepare the cells as described above in **PART I**.
2. Add 100 μl cells (1.5×10^5 cells/ml) to each well (i.e. 1.5×10^4 cells/well).
3. Incubate the plates for 18–20 hours at 37 °C in 5% CO_2. To ensure the even distribution of heat and CO_2, only stack plates 4–5 high in the incubator.

Fixation of plate(s)

Fix the plates as described in **PART I**.

Part III: ELISA

Addition of primary antibody

1. After fixation of the plates, wash them 3 times with wash buffer. Fill the wells completely with the wash buffer for each wash (approximately 300 μl per well).
2. Dilute antibodies (anti-influenza A NP monoclonal) 1:1000 or at optimal concentration (determined by earlier testing) in antibody diluent.
3. Add diluted antibody to each well (100 μl/well).
4. Cover plate(s) and incubate for 1 hour at room temperature.

Addition of secondary antibody

1. Wash plate(s) 3 times with wash buffer.
2. Dilute antibody (goat anti-mouse IgG; HRP-conjugated) 1:2000 or at optimal concentration (determined by earlier testing) in antibody diluent.
3. Add diluted antibody to each well (100 μl/well).
4. Cover plate(s) and incubate for 1 hour at room temperature.

Addition of substrate

1. Wash plate(s) 5 times with wash buffer.
2. Add freshly prepared substrate (10 mg OPD to each 20 ml citrate buffer + H_2O_2) to each well (100 μl/well).
3. Incubate for 5–10 minutes (or until colour change in VC is intense and before CC begins to change colour) at room temperature. Incubation time will vary between viruses.
4. Add stop solution (100 μl/well) to all wells.
5. Read the absorbance of the wells at 490 nm (OD_{490}).

Data analysis

1. Calculations are determined for each plate individually.
2. Determine the virus neutralization antibody 50% titre of each serum using the following equation:

$$x = \frac{(\text{average OD of VC wells}) - (\text{average OD of CC wells})}{2}$$

where x is the OD value at which 50% of the MDCK cells were infected.
All values **below or equal to** x are positive for neutralization activity. The reciprocal serum dilution corresponding to that well is the 50% neutralization antibody titre for

that serum sample. Serum dilutions are: well A 1:10; well B 1:20; well C 1:40; well D 1:80; well E 1:160; well F 1:320; well G 1:640; and well H 1:1280.

3. The cell control should have an $OD_{490}<0.2$. The virus control should have an $OD_{490}>0.8$.
4. The virus test dose (100x TCID) is confirmed by virus back titration. In most cases, the test dose of virus is acceptable if the back titration is positive in the 5–7 wells containing the lowest dilutions of test virus.
5. The serum positive controls should give titres within 2-fold of the values obtained in previous tests. The OD_{490} of the negative serum control should be similar to that observed for the virus control.

Occasionally, the microneutralization test may be difficult to interpret. In such cases, consider the factors presented in **TABLE 2.G-4**.

TABLE 2.G-4
Problems associated with interpretation of the microneutralization test

Problem	Possible cause(s)	Solution(s)
Weak or no colour in virus control wells	Problem with ELISA:	
	a. Wrong antibodies or substrate used	a. Check antibodies and substrate
	b. Buffer solutions incorrect	b. Prepare fresh buffers
	c. Test dose of virus too weak or no virus added to virus control wells	c. Redetermine virus TCID or adjust the dilution of virus used, ensuring virus is added to virus control cells
	d. Virus inactivated during virus-serum incubation step	d. Check incubator temperature and CO_2 level
	e. MDCK cells not optimal – e.g. too old (>30 passages); not in log-phase growth; or contaminated	e. Thaw a new vial of cells; do not allow cells to enter stationary phase
Weak or no neutralization by positive control sera	a. Test dose of virus too strong	a. Redetermine virus TCID or adjust the dilution of virus used
	b. Serum deteriorated	b. Obtain new antisera; and check storage conditions
	c. Cells not in optimal condition or passage level too high	c. Thaw a new vial of cells; do not allow cells to enter stationary phase
Neutralization by negative control sera	a. Nonspecific reaction or cross-reactivity	a. Heat-inactivate serum (56 °C for 30 minutes); check RDE treatment of animal serum; check samples for cross-reactive antibodies by testing against different subtypes; and try alternative serum treatment such as trypsin-heat-periodate
	b. Test dose of virus too weak	b. Redetermine virus TCID or adjust the dilution of virus used
Nonspecific virus inactivation	a. Serum not heat inactivated or contains nonspecific viral inhibitors	a. Heat-inactivate human serum (56 °C for 30 minutes) – treat animal serum with RDE
Monolayer toxicity	b. Serum not heat inactivated or is toxic to cells	b. Heat-inactivate serum – run serum toxicity check on MDCK cells and check microscopically for toxicity

Determination of cell count and viability

1. Trypsinize MDCK cells (as described above in **PART I, Preparation of MDCK cells for use in microneutralization assay**). Wash cells in PBS and resuspend in a small volume of media diluent (approximately 3–5 ml per flask) using a pipette.
2. Clean the haemacytometer thoroughly with 70% ethanol and dry with a lens tissue or soft lint-free cloth. Clean and dry the coverslip in the same way and press it gently on to the haemacytometer so that it adheres to and covers the counting area.
3. Place 100 µl of the cell suspension in one well of a 96-well microtitre plate.
4. Add 180 µl PBS to adjacent wells (2–3 wells will be sufficient).
5. Add 20 µl of trypan blue stain to an adjacent well.
6. Perform 10-fold serial dilutions with the cell suspension (from step **1**) until no cloudiness can be seen:
   — mix the cell suspension thoroughly with the Pipetman and transfer 20 µl to the well containing 180 µl diluent; and
   — perform 10-fold serial dilutions by transferring 20 µl suspension to 180 µl diluent. Mix 20 µl of diluted sample with 20 µl trypan blue stain and add mixture to the counting chamber of the haemacytometer. This is done by loading the Pipetman with the suspension (approximately 10 µl) and bringing it to the edge of the space immediately beneath the coverslip and injecting the mixture slowly until the chamber is full (do not overfill).
7. Count the cells immediately under the 10x objective of the microscope. Trypan blue will be absorbed by dead cells but not by viable cells – dead cells stain blue; viable cells are clear. Count the cells in each of the large corner quadrants (each quadrant consists of the 16 smaller squares marked in bold in **FIGURE 2.E-1** of **SECTION 2.E**).
8. After counting, rinse chamber and coverslip with 70% ethanol and dry.
9. Calculate the percentage viable cell concentration using the formula $C = n \times v^{-1}$ where:
   — C = the number of cells/ml;
   — n = the total number of viable cells counted; and
   — v^{-1} = volume (in ml) in each quadrant counted ($v-1$ = 0.1 mm depth x 1 mm^2 area = 0.1 mm^3 or 1×10^{-4} ml). For an example of how to determine this percentage see **BOX 2.G-1**.

BOX 2.G-1

Example of determining the percentage cell viability in a cell suspension diluted 1:10 in PBS and 1:2 in trypan blue stain

1. Count the number of viable and nonviable cells in each corner quadrant as in the example below:

Corner quadrant	No. of viable cells	No. of nonviable cells (stained with trypan blue)
1	106	0
2	88	2
3	99	0
4	115	1
Total	408	3

2. The average viable cell count (since 4 quadrants were counted) is 102 (408 divided by 4).

3. The volume of cell suspension counted is 0.1 mm³. Therefore, the concentration of cells in the suspension counted is:

$$\frac{102}{0.1 \text{ mm}^3} = \frac{102}{10^{-4} \text{ ml}} = (102 \times 10^4)/\text{ml} = 1.02 \times 10^6 \text{ cells/ml}$$

4. As the suspension was diluted from the original material 10-fold and diluted 2-fold in dye, the above result must be multiplied by 20 (i.e. 10¹ and 2) as follows:

$1.02 \times 10^6 \times 10^1 \times 2 = 2.04 \times 10^7$ cells/ml

5. The condensed version of the derivation of the equation is:

$$\frac{\text{viable cell count}}{4} \times 10^1 \times 2 \times (1 \times 10^4) = \text{number of viable cells/ml}$$

- 4 = the number of quadrants counted
- 10^1 = the dilution factor for PBS – if multiple 10-fold dilutions were made adjust accordingly
- 2 = the dilution factor for stain
- 1×10^4 = the volume counted per quadrant (per ml)

6. Percentage cell viability is then determined by the following equation:

$$\text{cell viability (\%)} = \frac{\text{number of viable cells counted}}{\text{total number of cells counted}} \times 100\%$$

In this example, cell viability $= \frac{408}{411} \times 100\% = 99.2\%$

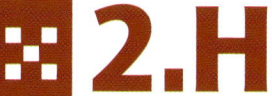

2.H
Identification of neuraminidase subtype by neuraminidase assay and neuraminidase inhibition test

The neuraminidase (NA) assay was initially described by Warren (1959) and later modified by Aymard-Henry et al. (1973). The principal steps involved in the NA assay are:

a. the release of free sialic acid from a fetuin substrate by the action of the NA enzyme of influenza viruses;
b. conversion of sialic acid to ß-formol pyruvic acid by periodate oxidation;
c. formation of a chromophore by thiobarbituric acid; and
d. extraction of the chromophore into an organic solvent for spectrophotometric analysis.

This method determines the potency of the viral NA and the standard NA dose for use in the NA inhibition (NAI) test. The principal steps in the NAI test then being:

a. incubation of the standardized NA dose with serial dilutions of test antisera, negative control serum and reference anti-NA serum;
b. determination of the inhibitory effect of sera on NA activity; and
c. calculation of the NAI titre.

Procedures for both the NA assay and NAI test are presented below.

Materials required
Equipment

Water-bath or incubator (37 °C)	Water-bath (100 °C)
Vortex mixer	Spectrophotometer

Supplies

Pipettes (1 ml) **BD Biosciences (Falcon) – cat. no. 357503**	Glass test-tubes (12 mm x 75 mm)
Pipettes (10 ml) **BD Biosciences (Falcon) – cat. no. 357530**	Racks for test-tubes
Multichannel pipetter **Rainin – cat. no. L12-200**	Tips for multichannel pipetter **Rainin – cat. no. RT-L200F**

Buffers and reagents

Periodate reagent (see below)	Arsenite reagent (see below)
2-thiobarbituric acid (2-TBA) reagent (see below)	Warrenoff reagent (see below)
Phosphate buffer (pH 5.8) (see below)	Fetuin **Sigma – cat. no. F3004**
Physiological saline (0.85% NaCl)	Water (distilled)

Preparation of solutions
Periodate reagent
- Dissolve 4.28 g sodium meta-periodate in 62 ml phosphoric acid and 32 ml distilled water. Mix well and store in glass.

Arsenite reagent (make up fresh each week)
- Dissolve 10 g sodium meta-arsenite and 7.1 g anhydrous sodium sulfate in 100 ml distilled water. Then add 0.3 ml concentrated sulfuric acid.

2-TBA reagent (make up fresh each week)
- Dissolve 1.2 g 2-TBA and 14.2 g anhydrous sodium sulfate in 200 ml distilled water by heating in a boiling water-bath.

Warrenoff reagent (make up fresh)
- Add 5 ml concentrated HCl in 100 ml of N-butanol.

Phosphate buffer (pH 5.8)
- Solution A – dissolve 9.08 g KH_2PO_4 in 1 litre distilled water.
- Solution B – dissolve 11.88 g Na_2HPO_4 in 1 litre distilled water.
- Working solution – mix 91.9 ml of solution A with 8.1 ml of solution B. Mix well, and if necessary adjust pH to 5.8 using solution A or solution B.

Fetuin (22 mg/ml)
- Dissolve 1 g fetuin in 45 ml distilled water.

Physiological saline (0.85% NaCl)
a. Prepare a 20x stock solution by dissolving 170 g NaCl in deionized distilled water to a total volume of 1 litre.
b. Sterilize by autoclaving.
c. To prepare physiological saline (0.85% NaCl) add 50ml 20x stock solution to 950 ml deionized distilled water.
d. Sterilize by autoclaving.
e. Store opened physiological saline at 4 °C for no longer than 3 weeks.

Procedure for neuraminidase (NA) assay
1. Make a serial 2-fold dilution of viral isolates in physiological saline (0.85% NaCl). For allantoic fluids, a suitable dilution series would be 1:2 to 1:128. If the virus has a higher level of NA activity, further dilutions may be needed. The positive control (reference virus) and unknown test viral isolates should be assayed in the same test. Set up two tubes as fetuin controls (i.e. tubes without virus but with all other reagents).
2. Transfer 50 μl of each virus dilution into each of a series of labelled test-tubes (12 mm x 75 mm). Include duplicate blank tubes that contain saline only.
3. To each test-tube (including the blanks) add 50 μl of a mixture of phosphate buffer (pH 5.8) and fetuin (mixed 1:1). Mix well and place at 37 °C for 18 hours.

4. Cool the test-tubes to 20 °C and add 50 µl periodate reagent to each tube. Mix thoroughly and place at room temperature for exactly 20 minutes.
5. Add 0.25 ml arsenite reagent. A brown colour will form resulting from the release of iodine. Shake until the brown colour disappears and then add 0.5 ml 2-TBA reagent. Mix thoroughly.
6. Immediately place the test-tubes safely in a boiling water-bath for 15 minutes. The red colour that develops indicates NA activity.
7. Cool the test-tubes to room temperature and add 1 ml Warrenoff reagent. Mix well using a vortex mixer or by vigorous shaking by hand. This will extract the colour into the organic (butanol) phase.
8. Centrifuge the test-tubes at 500 rpm for 5 minutes. At this stage, the upper (butanol) layer should be free of turbidity. If it has a misty appearance (due to the presence of water droplets) place the test-tubes in warm water (30 °C) until it becomes clear. Carefully pipette the upper phase into a colorimeter tube.
9. Read the optical density (OD) at 549 nm. Fetuin blanks are used to equilibrate the machine, and tests are read against the mean of the two fetuin blanks.
10. Record the results in the record sheet provided in **ANNEX VIII**. Determine the virus working dilution that gives an OD_{549} of 0.45 to 0.85.

Procedure for neuraminidase inhibition (NAI) test

1. Standardize antigens – dilute viruses to the working dilution determined above (i.e. the dilution giving OD_{549} readings of 0.45 to 0.85 after 18 hours incubation with fetuin in the NA assay).
2. Prepare serial 4-fold dilutions (i.e. 1:10; 1:40; 1:160; etc.) or half-log dilutions (i.e. 1:10; 1:32; 1:100; etc.) of serum. Transfer 50 µl of each serum dilution into a series of labelled test-tubes (12 mm x 75 mm). Add 50 µl of standardized virus to the serum and mix. Control and blank test-tubes should be included.
3. The neutralization reaction is carried out at 37 °C for 1 hour.
4. To each test-tube (including the blanks) add 50 µl of the mixture of phosphate buffer (pH 5.8) and fetuin (mixed 1:1); shake the test-tubes well and incubate at 37 °C for 18 hours.
5. Remove the test-tubes and assay for residual NA activity by adding the reagents as described in the procedure for the NA assay above (steps **4–9**).
6. Record the results in the record sheet provided in **ANNEX VIII**.
7. The essential reactions of the NAI test used for the antigenic characterization of unknown viral isolates are summarized in **TABLE 2.H-1**.

Interpretation of results

The NAI titre of an antiserum is defined as the dilution giving 50% inhibition of NA activity (NAI_{50}). In practice, this is determined by plotting the OD_{549} values against serum dilution using standard graph paper. The NAI_{50} titre is read from the graph as the serum dilution giving a 50% reduction in the OD_{549} value compared to the appropriate control test-tube (i.e. virus + negative control serum at the correct dilution).

An alternative method of calculating NAI titres is to divide the OD_{549} result for virus + diluted test serum by the OD_{549} result obtained for virus + negative control serum at the

TABLE 2.H-1
Essential elements of the NAI test used for the antigenic characterization of unknown viral isolates

Reaction	Reference anti-NA serum[a]	Negative control serum[b]	Fetuin-phosphate buffer	Viral isolate	Saline
Reference virus (test)	50 µl	–	50 µl	50 µl	–
Unknown virus (test)	50 µl	–	50 µl	50 µl	–
Reference virus (control)	–	50 µl	50 µl	50 µl	–
Unknown virus (control)	–	50 µl	50 µl	50 µl	–
Fetuin control	–	–	50 µl	–	100 µl

[a] 4-fold dilutions or half-log dilutions. Reference anti-NA serum can be any antiserum raised against a known influenza virus or concentrated NA.
[b] Dilution of 1:10 to 1:1000. Negative control serum is any normal serum to the same species as the anti-NA serum.

same dilution and multiply by 100 to obtain activity as a percentage. The percentage activity is plotted against serum dilution using standard graph paper. The NAI_{50} titre is read as that dilution which reduces NA activity by 50%. An example of the steps involved in this method of calculation is provided in **ANNEX VIII**.

If cross-reactivity between different antisera occurs with some viral isolates, identification of the isolate should be based on a 4-fold or greater difference in NAI titre. An example of NAI test results with their interpretation is shown in **TABLE 2.H-2**.

TABLE 2.H-2
Example of NAI test results for influenza A viruses

Test-tube no.	Control antigens	Reference sera[a,b]									Interpretation
		N1	N2	Nav2 (N3)	Nav4 (N4)	Nav5 (N5)	Nav2 (N6)	Neq1 (N7)	Neq2 (N8)	Neg	
1	A(N1)	3200	10	–	–	–	–	–	–	<10	–
2	A(N2)	<10	1600	–	–	–	–	–	–	<10	–
3	A(N3)	–	–	3200	–	–	–	–	–	<10	–
4	A(N4)	–	–	–	12 800	–	–	–	–	<10	–
5	A(N5)	–	–	–	–	6400	–	–	–	<10	–
6	A(N6)	–	–	–	–	–	12 800	–	–	<10	–
7	A(N7)	–	–	–	–	–	–	12 800	–	<10	–
8	A(N8)	–	–	–	–	–	–	–	3200	<10	–
9	Field isolate 1	<10	1600	<10	<10	<10	<10	<10	<10	<10	A(N2)

[a] All reference antisera are goat antisera from the United States National Institutes of Health.
[b] The values shown are NAI titres.
Neg: negative control serum (uninfected serum).

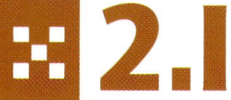

2.1
Molecular identification of influenza isolates

Since 1977, two influenza type A subtypes – A(H3N2) and A(H1N1) – have co-circulated in human populations. In 2009, a novel and highly transmissible A(H1N1) influenza virus was detected in humans and subsequently caused an influenza pandemic. Two antigenically and genetically distinct lineages of influenza B viruses[1] are also currently circulating among humans. Such complex co-circulation of multiple types and subtypes of influenza viruses increases the difficulty of diagnosis and virus identification. Routine methods for diagnosing influenza infection (including virus culture and antigen detection) are both sensitive and specific. However, molecular techniques to directly detect influenza A or B genetic material in respiratory samples or viral cultures can greatly facilitate the investigation of outbreaks of respiratory illness. In addition, such techniques can also be highly useful in the rapid identification of human influenza A subtypes, including those with the potential to cause a pandemic.

Molecular assays should be used, in conjunction with other diagnostic assays and clinical and epidemiological information, to:

- detect influenza virus type A or B in symptomatic patients from viral RNA in respiratory specimens and virus culture;
- determine the subtype of human influenza A viruses;
- presumptively identify virus in patient respiratory specimens or viral cultures which may be infected with influenza A of subtype H5 (Asian lineage); and
- detect potentially novel or newly evolving influenza A viruses.

Acceptable materials for use with molecular techniques include extracted viral RNA from human respiratory specimens (such as nasopharyngeal swabs and aspirates, oropharyngeal aspirates or washes, throat swabs, sputum, tracheal aspirates or broncheoalveolar lavage) or viral culture. Swab specimens should be collected using swabs with a synthetic tip (such as polyester or Dacron®) and an aluminium or plastic shaft, and should be submitted in viral transport medium (see **SECTION 2.A**). Swabs with cotton tips and wooden shafts are not recommended. Specimens collected with swabs made of calcium alginate are not acceptable.

Specimens should be transported to the laboratory from the collection site with a coolant to maintain a refrigerated temperature of approximately 2–8 °C. Specimens should not be frozen except for those sent from remote locations. Specimens should be inoculated for culturing and put into lysis buffer within 72 hours of collection in all cases except for those collected at remote facilities. Any specimens that are frozen upon receipt or are

---

[1] B/Sichuan/379/99 (B/Yamagata/16/88-lineage) and B/Shandong/7/97 (B/Victoria/2/87-lineage).

at elevated temperatures should be noted. Specimens added to nucleic acid extraction lysis buffer according to recommended procedures can be considered to be non-infectious and handled under BSL-2 precautions and practice. Specimens may be rejected if they are not kept at 2–4°C (for ≤4 days) or frozen at -70 °C or below – or if they are incompletely labelled or documented.

Specimen processing should be performed in accordance with pertaining national biological safety regulations. Manipulation of human respiratory samples should be performed under BSL-2 containment. Manipulation of samples from patients meeting clinical and epidemiological risk factors that suggest possible infection with A/H5N1 highly pathogenic avian influenza virus should be performed at a ***minimum*** of BSL-2 containment and BSL-3 practices. All manipulations of live virus samples must be performed within a class-II (or higher) biosafety cabinet. Clinical specimens from humans and from animals should ***never*** be processed in the same laboratory. However they can be processed in the same institution if the separation of working rooms for animal and human specimens is clear and strict. This is to eliminate the risk of cross contamination of human and animal samples.

Conventional and real-time reverse-transcription polymerase chain reaction

Polymerase chain reaction (PCR) is a technique used to amplify specific regions of DNA from very low levels of starting template DNA. Reverse-transcription PCR (RT-PCR) is an extension of this technique in which template RNA is first reverse-transcribed into complementary DNA (cDNA) (**BOX 2.I-1**). This cDNA then undergoes amplification by PCR.

In addition, a number of methods have been designed that use fluorescent dyes to detect or quantitate in real time the amplification of DNA by PCR. Several such real-time RT-PCR (rRT-PCR) methods involve the use of SYBR® green, which binds to double-stranded DNA and fluoresces when excited by light of the appropriate wavelength. Although SYBR® green will detect amplification of DNA, all amplified products (both desired and nonspecific) will fluoresce, making it difficult to determine if the amplified DNA is the specifically intended product. Other methods incorporate a labelled oligonucleotide probe (such as a TaqMan® probe) that is dually labelled with a fluorescent label (or fluorophore) and a quencher dye. In this case, because the probe binds to the specific target and does not bind to nonspecific products, fluorescence is only observed if the target is amplified.

A number of other methods have also been designed using for example "minor groove binding" probes, FRET probes, Molecular Beacons, and Scorpion probes that also allow the detection of amplified specific targets on a real-time basis. However, it is important to note that, as with conventional RT-PCR, the sensitivity and specificity of real-time systems are directly dependent upon the quality of the oligonucleotide primers used for amplification of the DNA target regions.

Since genetic sequences differ among different types and subtypes of influenza viruses, it is possible to design PCR primers and probes that will differentially detect only one influenza type or subtype. Genes that encode the internal virus proteins such as the M1 matrix protein or the non-structural NS_1 protein are highly conserved among influenza viruses and are thus useful targets for the universal detection and differentiation of type A and type B influenza viruses. Because influenza A subtypes are defined by their surface HA and NA proteins, primers that specifically amplify the corresponding genes are effective for determining the subtype of influenza A viruses. The emergence of human cases of influenza A(H5N1) in some countries highlights the need for highly sensitive, accurate and rapid diagnostic assays that can be used in surveillance to detect the spread of influenza viruses and to aid in public health planning, preparedness and response. Similarly, a number of protocols have been designed for the detection of influenza B viruses based on their NS gene.

In this manual, both conventional RT-PCR and real-time RT-PCR are outlined for the detection and characterization of influenza viruses. However, the procedures for nucleic acid extraction and analysis included below are for illustrative purposes only. Specific procedures and protocols are subject to change. Reference should be made to the WHO web site or to a WHO Collaborating Centre for the most current guidance. For example, updated real-time PCR methods and conventional PCR assays for the detection and characterization of pandemic (H1N1) 2009 influenza viruses were made available on the WHO web site,[1] as was the corresponding CDC protocol.[2]

Disclaimer: Although the names of vendors or manufacturers are provided as examples of suitable product sources, their inclusion does not imply endorsement by the World Health Organization.

BOX 2.I-1

Principles of RT-PCR

PCR and RT-PCR methods have been designed for the detection and characterization of a number of different infectious agents including bacteria and viruses. Because the genome of influenza viruses consists of eight single-stranded RNA segments, RT-PCR is necessary for the amplification of specific influenza gene targets. RT-PCR can be used for the detection of influenza viruses in respiratory samples taken from patients with influenza-like illness or for the characterization of viruses grown in cell culture or embryonated eggs.

Conventional RT-PCR reactions typically require a pair of oligonucleotides (known as primers), four deoxyribonucleoside triphosphates (dNTPs), template RNA, reverse transcriptase and Taq DNA polymerase. Following reverse transcription of the RNA target to cDNA, the cDNA is subjected to repeated thermal cycling. In the case of conventional RT-PCR this causes template denaturation (at 95 °C), primer annealing (at 45–60 °C) and product extension (at 72 °C). For some assays and for real-time RT-PCR, product extension at 72 °C is not necessary. Taq DNA polymerase is DNA-dependent and thermostable, and is therefore not inactivated during the denaturation steps and does not need to be replaced at every round of the amplification cycle. Because the products of one round of amplification serve as templates for the next, each successive cycle essentially doubles the amount of the desired DNA product. The recent availability of improved "one-step" RT-PCR strategies have decreased the number of pipetting steps required, making the process technically easier and less susceptible to contamination.

---

[1] www.who.int/csr/resources/publications/swineflu/diagnostic_recommendations/en/index.html
[2] www.who.int/csr/resources/publications/swineflu/realtimeptpcr/en/index.html

Materials required
Equipment

Thermocycler (for conventional RT-PCR); Real-time thermocycler (for real-time RT-PCR)	Microcentrifuge (adjustable up to 13 000 rpm)
Electrophoresis power supply for conventional RT-PCR	Ultraviolet light source for conventional RT-PCR (preferably at 302 nm wavelength; but sources at 250–310 nm can be used)
Agarose gel casting tray and electrophoresis chamber for conventional RT-PCR	Vortex mixer

Supplies

96-well 0.2 ml PCR reaction tube strips or PCR reaction plates	8-well strip caps for conventional RT-PCR, or 8-well optical strip caps for real-time RT-PCR
Sterile nuclease-free 1.5 ml microcentrifuge tubes	Cooler racks for 1.5 ml microcentrifuge tubes and 96-well 0.2ml PCR reaction plates
Sterile pipette tips (RNase-free with aerosol barrier)	Adjustable micropipettes (10–1000 µl)
Disposable powder-free gloves	Laboratory marking pen

Buffers, reagents and media

RNA extraction kit	Forward and reverse oligonucleotide primers
Positive control viral RNAs – A(H1N1); A(H3N2) and B	One-step quantitative RT-PCR probe hydrolysis kit (real-time RT-PCR) or one-step RT-PCR kit (conventional RT-PCR)
Oligonucleotide hydrolysis probes labelled with flourophore (e.g. FAM) and quencher (e.g. BHQ-1) for real-time RT-PCR	Molecular-grade sterile distilled H2O (RNase and DNase free) for RT-PCR reaction set-up
Molecular-grade 99% ethanol (RNase and DNase free)	Molecular weight markers for electrophoresis of RT-PCR products for conventional RT-PCR
10x stock tris-borate-EDTA (TBE) buffer (see below) for conventional RT-PCR	Agarose for electrophoresis of RT-PCR products (see below) for conventional RT-PCR
Ethidium bromide (10 mg/ml) for agarose gel preparation for conventional RT-PCR	6x xylene cyanol gel loading buffer without bromophenol blue (see below) for conventional RT-PCR **Sigma – cat. no. X4126**
DNAzap **Ambion – cat. no. AM9890**	RNase away **Invitrogen – cat. no. 10328011**
5% bleach for decontamination	70% ethanol for disinfecting/cleaning purposes
Deionized H$_2$O for buffer and agarose gel preparation	

Preparation of media, reagents and buffers for conventional RT-PCR

10x tris-borate-EDTA (TBE) buffer

a. Dissolve 108 g of tris(hydroxymethyl)aminomethane (tris Base), 55 g of boric acid and 20 ml of 0.5M EDTA in slightly less than 1 litre of water.
b. Adjust the volume to 1 litre by adding water.
c. If white clumps begin to precipitate in the solution, place the bottle in hot water until the clumps dissolve.
d. Check the pH – if outside the range of 8.3 ± 0.3 prepare the solution again. **Note: do NOT adjust the pH, as a change in ion concentration will affect the migration of the DNA through the gel**.

There is no need to sterilize the solution, which can be stored at room temperature.

For use as a 1x TBE buffer (working buffer), dilute the 10x stock 10-fold (i.e. 100 ml 10x TBE in 900 ml water). Commercially available concentrated TBE may be 5x or 20x and should be diluted accordingly.

1 or 2% agarose

1% agarose gels should be used for larger PCR products (approximately 500 to 1200 base pairs, while 2% agarose gels should be used for smaller PCR products (under 500 base pairs). Add 1 or 2 g of agarose respectively to 100 ml 1x TBE heated in a hot water-bath or microwave until dissolved. Allow to cool slightly and add ethidium bromide at a final concentration of 0.5 µg/ml.

6x xylene cyanol gel loading buffer without bromophenol blue

a. Dissolve 4 g of sucrose and 25 mg xylene cyanol in slightly less than 10 ml of water. Adjust the volume to 10 ml by adding water.
b. Store at 4 °C to avoid mould growing in the sucrose. Loading buffer will last for several years.
c. For use as a 1x loading buffer, add the appropriate amount to the DNA sample before loading onto the gel – e.g. 5 µl of loading buffer to 25 µl DNA sample.

Conventional and real-time RT-PCR

Note: the procedures described here assume a basic familiarity with nucleic acid handling techniques as well as conventional and real-time RT-PCR techniques.

General precautions

Due to the sensitivity of RT-PCR based assays, special precautions must be followed to avoid false-positive amplifications. The following precautionary steps are recommended:

1. Maintain separate areas for assay setup and for handling nucleic acids.
2. Maintain separate dedicated equipment (e.g. pipettes; microcentrifuges) and supplies (e.g. microcentrifuge tubes; pipette tips) for assay setup and for handling nucleic acids.
3. Wear a clean laboratory coat and powder-free disposable gloves (not previously worn) when setting up assays.
4. Change gloves between work areas and whenever contamination is suspected.

5. Work surfaces, pipettes and centrifuges should be cleaned and decontaminated with cleaning products such as 5% bleach, DNAzap or RNase away to minimize the risk of nucleic acid contamination. Residual bleach should be removed using 70% ethanol.
6. Turn on the thermocycler and (for conventional PCR) the ultraviolet light source, and allow the systems to warm up for 30 minutes before use.
7. Always check the expiry date of reagents prior to use. Do not use expired reagent.
8. Reagents, master mix and RNA should be maintained on a cold block or on ice during preparation and use to ensure stability.
9. Thaw the master-mix vial. Do not refreeze. Store at 4 °C.
10. Mix the master mix by inversion.
11. Vortex all primers and probes.
12. Spin all primers, probes and reagents for 30 seconds and then place on ice.
13. Keep reagent and reaction tubes capped or covered as much as possible.

Golden rule: In terms of Good Laboratory Practise clinical specimens from humans and from animals should **never** be processed in the same laboratory. However they could be processed in the same institution if the separation of working rooms for animal and human specimens is clear and strictly observed. This is to eliminate the risk of cross contamination of human and animal samples. (http://www.hpa-standardmethods.org.uk/documents/qsop/pdf/qsop38.pdf)

Viral RNA extraction

The performance of RT-PCR amplification based assays depends upon the amount and quality of sample template RNA. A number of commercially available extraction procedures have been shown to generate highly purified RNA when following the manufacturer's recommended procedures. RNA-extraction procedures should be qualified and validated for recovery and purity before testing specimens.

1. Extract viral RNA from the clinical specimen(s) using an appropriate extraction kit in accordance with the manufacturer's instructions.
2. Use viral RNA immediately in real-time or conventional RT-PCR – or aliquot into small volumes and freeze at -70 °C until use.

Quality control

Quality-control procedures are intended to monitor reagent and assay performance. Test all positive controls prior to running diagnostic samples with each new reagent kit lot to ensure all reagents and components are working properly. Good laboratory practice recommends including a positive RNA extraction control (EC) in each nucleic acid isolation batch for each run. The EC provides a secondary negative control that validates the nucleic extraction procedure and reagent integrity.

Each sample RNA extract is tested by separate primer sets. Negative template controls (NTCs) and positive template controls (PTCs) for all primer/probe sets should be included in each run. The human RNase P gene (RNP) primer and probe set serves as an internal positive control for human RNA. Reaction assay mixtures are made as master mix cocktails and dispensed into a PCR reaction plate or strip tube that meets the manufacturer's requirements and specifications for the PCR platform being used. Extracted nucleic acid,

PTCs or sterile distilled water (RNase and DNase free) is then added to the appropriate test reactions and controls.

Test procedure
Reagent preparation
Note: keep all reagents on cold rack during assay set up.

Primers[1]
a. Thaw frozen aliquots of primers.
b. Vortex all primers.
c. Briefly centrifuge all primers and then place in cold rack.

RT-PCR reagents
a. Place reagents in cold rack.
b. Thaw any frozen reagents and mix by inversion.
c. Briefly centrifuge reagents and place in cold rack.

RT-PCR test procedure
Note: all reactions should be carried out on ice.

1. Label one 1.5 ml microcentrifuge tube for each primer/probe set.
2. Determine the number of reactions (N) to set up per assay. It is necessary to make excess reaction cocktail for the EC, NTC and PTC reactions and to allow for pipetting error.
   — If the number of samples (n) including controls is 1–14, then N = n + 1.
   — If the number of samples (n) including controls is >15, then N = n + 2.
3. The master mix components for both conventional and real-time RT-PCR are indicated below. The specific volumes and components used may differ depending on assay design and the source of commercial reagents. Assay-specific recommendations should be followed in all cases.

Conventional RT-PCR master mix	Real-time RT-PCR master mix
Nuclease-free water	Nuclease-free water
Forward primer	Forward primer
Reverse primer	Reverse primer
dNTPs	Fluorescent probe
Enzyme mix	Enzyme mix
Reaction mix	Reaction mix

4. In the assay set-up area, dispense reaction mixtures into the labelled 1.5 ml microcentrifuge tubes. After addition of the water, mix by pipetting up and down. Do **not** vortex.
5. Centrifuge for 5 seconds to collect the contents on the bottom of the tube then place the tube in a cold rack.
6. Set up reaction strip tubes or plates in a 96-well cooler rack.

---

[1] It is recommended that laboratories that have concerns about identifying currently circulating viruses should contact a WHOCC for assistance in identifying the optimal primers to be used.

7. Add 20 µl of each master mix into each well, going across the rows. An example of the setting up of test and sample plates is shown in **TABLE 2.I-1**.
8. Before moving the plate to the nucleic acid handling area, set up the NTC reactions in column 1 in the assay set-up area. Pipette 5 µl nuclease-free water into the NTC wells (the reaction volume is then 25 µl). Cap the NTC wells.
9. Cover the plate and move it to the nucleic acid handling area.
10. Vortex the tubes containing the samples for 5 seconds.
11. Centrifuge the tubes for 5 seconds.
12. Set up the extracted nucleic acid sample reactions in the cold rack. As shown in **TABLE 2.I-1** samples can be added by column. Pipette 5 µl of the first sample into all the wells labelled for that sample (e.g. sample 1 (S1)). Change tips after each single addition.
13. Cap the wells of each column once the sample has been added. This will help to prevent sample cross contamination and enable sample addition to be clearly tracked.
14. Change gloves when necessary to avoid contamination.
15. Repeat steps **12–14** for the remaining samples.
16. Add 5 µl of mock extracted sample to the EC wells (column 11). Cap the EC wells.
17. Pipette 5 µl PTC RNA into all the appropriate wells (column 12). Cap the PTC wells once this is done.
18. Centrifuge tube strips in a flash centrifuge for 10–15 seconds. Return strip tubes to cold rack. If using plates, centrifuge at 2000 rpm for 30 seconds at 4 °C. Return plates to the cold rack.

TABLE 2.I-1
Example of set up of plates for tests and samples
Test set-up

Row	Column											
	1	2	3	4	5	6	7	8	9	10	11	12
A	FluA	FluA	FluA	FluA	FluA	FluA	FluA	FluA	FluA	FluA	FluA	FluA
B	H1	H1	H1	H1	H1	H1	H1	H1	H1	H1	H1	H1
C	H3	H3	H3	H3	H3	H3	H3	H3	H3	H3	H3	H3
D	FluB	FluB	FluB	FluB	FluB	FluB	FluB	FluB	FluB	FluB	FluB	FluB
E	RNP	RNP	RNP	RNP	RNP	RNP	RNP	RNP	RNP	RNP	RNP	RNP
F	-	-	-	-	-	-	-	-	-	-	-	-
G	-	-	-	-	-	-	-	-	-	-	-	-
H	-	-	-	-	-	-	-	-	-	-	-	-

Additional tests can be added for the identification of other subtypes including H5N1 and pandemic (H1N1) 2009.

Sample set-up

Row	Column											
	1	2	3	4	5	6	7	8	9	10	11	12
A	NTC	S1	S2	S3	S4	S5	S6	S7	S8	S9	EC	PTC
B	NTC	S1	S2	S3	S4	S5	S6	S7	S8	S9	EC	PTC
C	NTC	S1	S2	S3	S4	S5	S6	S7	S8	S9	EC	PTC
D	NTC	S1	S2	S3	S4	S5	S6	S7	S8	S9	EC	PTC
E	NTC	S1	S2	S3	S4	S5	S6	S7	S8	S9	EC	PTC
F	-	-	-	-	-	-	-	-	-	-	-	-
G	-	-	-	-	-	-	-	-	-	-	-	-
H	-	-	-	-	-	-	-	-	-	-	-	-

Negative template controls (NTCs) should be added first (to column 1) before any of the samples (S1–S9) are added to check for any contamination of the master mix. EC should be added (column 11) after the samples have been added to check for cross contamination during sample preparation or addition. PTCs should be added last (to column 12) after all the samples have been added and after all the wells containing samples and NTCs have been sealed.

Thermocycler or real-time PCR systems should be programmed in accordance with the assay-specific recommendations. The actual temperature and time parameters to be used will depend upon the specific chemistry and assay design.

Conventional RT-PCR amplification conditions

Reaction step	Temperature	Time
Reverse transcription	42–50 °C	30 minutes
RT inactivation/Taq activation	95 °C	2–15 minutes

PCR amplification (35–45 cycles)
  Denaturation
  Primer annealing
  Template extension
	
	95 °C
	45–60 °C[a]
	72 °C
		
		15 seconds
		30 seconds
		30–120 seconds[b]

Hold	4 °C	hold

[a] Primer annealing temperature will depend upon the specific assay used.
[b] Template extension at 72 °C may not be necessary for all assay designs.

Real-time RT-PCR amplification conditions

Reaction step	Temperature	Time
Reverse transcription	42–50 °C[a]	30 minutes
RT inactivation/Taq activation	95 °C	2–15 minutes

PCR amplification (35–45 cycles)
  Denaturation
  Primer annealing/Template extension
	
	95 °C
	45–60 °C[b]
		
		15 seconds
		5–60 seconds

[a] Specific temperature and time parameters depend upon the specific chemistry and assay design used.
[b] Fluorescence data should be collected during the Primer annealing/Template extension step.

Interpretation of results
Conventional RT-PCR

Electrophoresis of all reactions including all test samples and controls must be performed on a 1 or 2% agarose gel (1x TBE) containing ethidium bromide at a final concentration of 0.5 μg/ml. Mix 10 μl of each reaction mixture with an equal volume of loading buffer containing 0.25% xylene cyanol (but not Bromphenol Blue as this may obscure the visualization of DNA fragments of 100–300 base pairs). Each agarose gel should include a DNA size standard range of 50–1000 base pairs. Standard gel electrophoresis should be performed at 100 V for 30 minutes.

NTC reactions for all primer sets should not exhibit the presence of amplified DNA products of similar size to that of the positive control reaction. If a false positive occurs with one or more of the primer NTC reactions, sample contamination may have occurred. Invalidate the run and repeat the assay with stricter adherence to the procedure guidelines.

PTC reactions should produce positive results with each reaction as demonstrated by the presence of amplified DNA products **of appropriate size**. If expected positive reactivity is not achieved, invalidate the run and repeat the assay with stricter adherence to procedure guidelines. Determine the cause of failed PTC reactivity and implement corrective actions, then document both the results of the investigation and the corrective actions taken. Do not use PTC reagents that do not generate the expected result.

The EC should **not** exhibit the presence of amplified DNA products of similar size to those of the PTC reactions. If any influenza-specific primer exhibits the presence of such products, interpret as follows:

- possible contamination of RNA-extraction reagents – invalidate the run and confirm the integrity of RNA-extraction reagents prior to further testing; and/or
- cross contamination of samples occurred during the RNA-extraction procedures or assay setup – invalidate the run and repeat the assay with stricter adherence to procedure guidelines.

All clinical samples should exhibit the presence of human gene DNA product, thus indicating the presence of sufficient human RNA showing that the specimen is of acceptable quality. However, it is possible that some samples may fail to give positive reactions due to low cell numbers in the original clinical sample. Failure to detect human RNA in any of the clinical samples may indicate:

- improper extraction of nucleic acid from clinical materials resulting in loss of RNA or carry-over of RT-PCR inhibitors from clinical specimens;
- insufficient human cellular material in the sample to enable detection;
- improper assay set up and execution; and/or
- reagent or equipment malfunction.

When all controls meet the stated requirements a specimen is considered presumptive positive for influenza A virus if the reaction "InfA" exhibits the presence of amplified DNA product of appropriate size. If the reaction for influenza A is positive, it should also be positive for a specific subtype (i.e. A(H1); pandemic A(H1); A(H3); A(H5) etc). A specimen is considered presumptive positive for a particular influenza A subtype if **both** the InfA and the respective subtype reaction exhibits the presence of amplified DNA product of the appropriate size.

When all controls meet the stated requirements, a specimen is considered presumptive positive for influenza B virus if the "InfB" reaction exhibits the presence of amplified DNA products of appropriate size.

When all controls meet the stated requirements, a specimen is considered negative for influenza virus if neither InfA nor InfB reactions exhibit the presence of amplified DNA products of appropriate size.

Real-time RT-PCR

After the run has completed, view the amplification plots. Confirm that the threshold is positioned so that it is close to but above the background signal and within the exponential phase of the fluorescence curves (**FIGURE 2.I-1**).

FIGURE 2.I-1
Real-time RT-PCR amplification plot

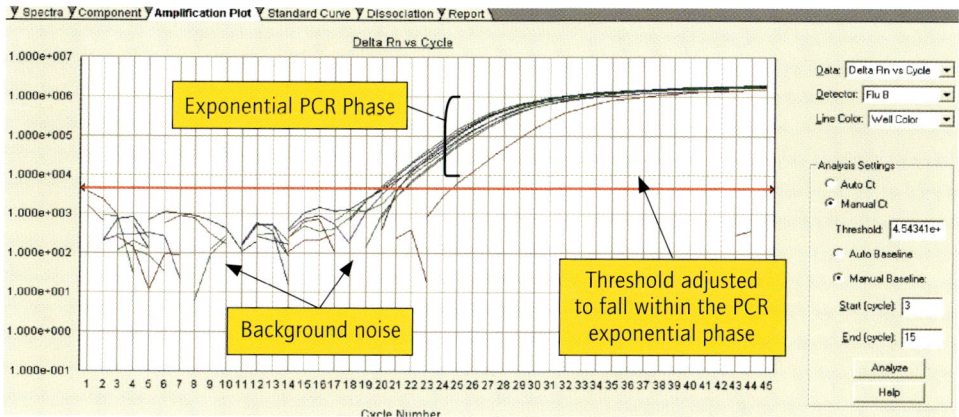

The NTC reactions for all primer sets should not exhibit the presence of amplified DNA products of size similar to that of the positive control reaction. If a false positive occurs with one or more of the primer NTC reactions, sample contamination may have occurred. Invalidate the run and repeat the assay with stricter adherence to the procedure guidelines.

PTC reactions should produce a positive result with each reaction as demonstrated by fluorescence growth curves that cross the threshold. If expected positive reactivity is not achieved, invalidate the run and repeat the assay with stricter adherence to procedure guidelines. Determine the cause of failed PTC reactivity and implement corrective actions, and then document both the results of the investigation and the corrective actions taken. Do not use PTC reagents that do not generate the expected result.

The EC should **not** exhibit fluorescence growth curves that cross the threshold line. If any influenza-specific primer/probes exhibit a growth curve that crosses the threshold line, interpret as follows:

- possible contamination of RNA-extraction reagents – invalidate the run and confirm the integrity of RNA-extraction reagents prior to further testing; and/or
- cross contamination of samples occurred during the RN- extraction procedures or assay setup – invalidate the run and repeat the assay with stricter adherence to procedure guidelines.

All clinical samples should exhibit a positive result with the human gene specific target as demonstrated by fluorescence growth curves that cross the threshold at or before 40 CT[1] (threshold cycle) thus indicating the presence of sufficient human RNA and indicating that the specimen is of acceptable quality. However, it is possible that some samples may fail to give positive reactions due to low cell numbers in the original clinical sample. Samples taken from animal (including avian) species or cell culture may exhibit either no human gene reaction or a weak reaction. Failure to detect human RNA in any of the clinical samples may indicate:

- improper extraction of nucleic acid from clinical materials resulting in loss of RNA or carry-over of RT-PCR inhibitors from clinical specimens;
- insufficient human cellular material in the sample to enable detection;
- improper assay set up and execution; and/or
- reagent or equipment malfunction.

In such cases, the cause should be investigated and corrective actions implemented and documented before repeating the assay.

When all controls meet the stated requirements (**TABLE 2.I-2**) a specimen is considered presumptive positive for influenza A virus if the reaction "InfA" exhibits a fluorescence growth curve that cross the threshold line. If the reaction for influenza A is positive, it should also be positive for a specific subtype (i.e. A(H1); pandemic A(H1); A(H3); A(H5) etc). A specimen is considered presumptive positive for an influenza A subtype if **both** the InfA and the respective subtype reaction exhibit a fluorescence growth curve that crosses the threshold line.

TABLE 2.I-2
Example of expected performance of control reactions

Control Type	Internal Control	Used to Monitor	InfA	InfB	H1	H3	Hum
Positive	PTC	Substantial reagent failure including primer and probe integrity	+	+	+	+	+
Negative	NTC	Reagent and/or environmental contamination	–	–	–	–	–
Extraction	EC	Failure in lysis and extraction procedure	–	–	–	–	+/–

---

[1] The CT value is defined as the PCR cycle at which a statistically significant increase in the fluorescence signal is first detected. CT values form the basis of quantitative comparisons of individual PCR reactions. The smaller the CT value, the larger the quantity of target cDNA in a given reaction.

When all controls meet the stated requirements, a specimen is considered presumptive positive for influenza B virus if the "InfB" reaction exhibits a fluorescence growth curve that crosses the threshold line.

When all controls meet the stated requirements, a specimen is considered negative for influenza virus if neither InfA nor InfB reactions exhibit fluorescence growth curves that cross the threshold line.

If the controls in the assay do not exhibit the expected performance as described above for both conventional and real-time RT-PCR, the assay may have been set up and/or executed improperly, or reagent or equipment malfunction could have occurred. Invalidate the run and retest. If a combination of results other than those shown in **TABLE 2.I-2** is generated, the result is invalid. Repeat extraction and retest the sample. If after repeat testing the result is unchanged, report the result as ***invalid***. For a general guide to the interpretation and reporting of results refer to **TABLE 2.I-3**.

TABLE 2.I-3
Guide for conventional and real-time RT-PCR results interpretation and reporting

InfA	InfB	H1	H3	2009 H1 (pandemic)	H5	Hum	Interpretation	Actions	Report
-	-	-	-	-	-	+	No influenza virus detected	Report	Influenza A or B Virus Not Detected
+	-	NA	NA	NA	NA	±	Influenza A	Report	Positive for Influenza A Virus
-	+	NA	NA	NA	NA	±	Influenza B	Report	Positive for Influenza B Virus
+	-	+	-	-	-	±	Influenza A/H1	Report	Positive for Influenza A/H1 Virus
+	-	-	+	-	-	±	Influenza A/H3	Report	Positive for Influenza A/H3 Virus
+	-	-	-	+	-	±	Influenza A/ 2009 H1 pdm	Report	Positive for Influenza A/ H1pdm Virus
-	+	-	-	-	-	±	Influenza B	Report	Positive for Influenza B Virus
+	-	-	-	-	-	±	Influenza A, no subtype result	Retest; Notify WHOCC	Inconclusive: Influenza A "unsubtypable" virus detected; potential novel strain
-	-	-	-	-	-	-	Inconclusive	Retest	Inconclusive
+	-	-	-	-	+	±	Influenza A/H5	Retest; Notify WHOCC	Presumptive Positive for AH5 Virus

NA = subtype markers are not tested in this scenario.

Limitations of both conventional and real-time RT-PCR

Negative results do not preclude influenza virus infection and should not be used as the sole basis for treatment or other management decisions. A false-negative may occur if:

- a specimen is improperly collected, transported or handled;
- amplification inhibitors or other interfering materials are present in the specimen;
- there is an inadequate number of viruses present in the specimen; or
- there is excess DNA or RNA template in the specimen – if a negative result is obtained and high levels of nucleic acid are suspected, the extracted sample can be tested at 2 or more dilutions (e.g. 1:10 and 1:100) to check the result.

Individuals who received nasally administered influenza A vaccine may have positive test results for up to three days after vaccination.

Positive and negative predictive values are also highly dependent on prevalence. False negatives are more likely during peak activity when the prevalence of disease is high. False positives are more likely during periods of low influenza activity when prevalence is moderate to low.

Children tend to shed virus more abundantly and for longer periods than adults. Therefore, specimens from adults may have lower sensitivity levels than specimens from children. Optimum specimen types and timing for peak viral levels during infections caused by a novel influenza A virus have not been determined. The collection of multiple specimens from the same patient may therefore be necessary to detect the virus.

If there is a mutation in the target region, a specific novel influenza A virus may not be detected or may be detected less predictably.

For these and other reasons, analysts need to be trained and familiar with testing procedures and interpretation of results, and reagents must not be used past their expiry date.

Additional methods for the molecular identification of influenza

In addition to gel electrophoresis for conventional RT-PCR and fluorescence detection by real-time RT-PCR, other methods of post-PCR amplification can be used to characterize PCR products such as Restriction Fragment Length Polymorphism (RFLP); hybridization to immobilized oligonucleotide probes; or genetic sequence analysis.

- **RFLP** – has been used successfully to identify genetic variants of seasonal influenza viruses. RFLP relies on the presence or absence of specific endonuclease restriction sites that allow amplified gene segments to be characterized based on the expected length of DNA fragments following endonuclease digestion.
- **Probe hybridization** – a number of commercial assays have been developed that utilize hybridization to specific oligonucleotide probes bound to immobilized surfaces such as a microarray chip or beads. Although these methods can be time consuming and expensive to perform, the ability to analyze several probes at the same time increases the amount of data.
- **Genetic sequence analysis** – determination of the specific genetic sequence of amplified DNA is the highest level of genetic characterization. Although these methods typically require more time and resources, genetic-sequence data allows for the detailed analysis necessary for evolutionary characterization as well as for the identification of specific mutations with biological significance, such as those leading to changes in antiviral resistance; antigenic variability; and pathogenicity in different hosts.

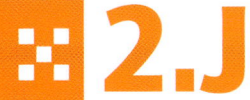

2.J
Virus identification by immunofluorescence antibody staining

Immunofluorescence antibody (IFA) staining of virus-infected cells in original clinical specimens and field isolates is a rapid and sensitive method for diagnosing respiratory and other viral infections. During recent years, monoclonal antibodies against several clinically important respiratory viruses have become commercially available and have been thoroughly evaluated in many laboratories. It is preferable for IFA staining to be performed on isolates rather than original clinical specimens. The use of isolates allows any virus that is present to be amplified for use in other studies.

However, where rapid diagnosis is needed, this procedure is often carried out on clinical specimens. Suitable clinical specimens are nasal swabs; throat swabs; nasopharyngeal aspirates; nasal wash; throat wash; transtracheal aspirates; and bronchoalveolar lavage fluids. To avoid the loss of virus-infected desquamated respiratory epithelial cells by lysis, specimens must be chilled immediately after collection and should be processed within 1–2 hours. The cells are washed in order to remove contaminating mucus and then spotted onto microscope slides, dried, fixed, stained and examined for specific intracellular staining of the antigen-antibody complex by fluorescence microscopy.

The sensitivity of the method is greatly influenced by the quality of the specimen; the specificity of the reagents used; and the level of experience of those performing, reading and interpreting the test. If possible, more than one slide should be prepared from each specimen just in case re-staining is required. Furthermore, a collection of slides from known positive specimens is the best source of positive controls for future assays.

Other rapid diagnostic tests for influenza

There are now a number of commercially available rapid diagnostic tests, for use in screening for influenza virus infections, which can provide results within 30 minutes. Most of these tests are immunoassays which detect influenza viral antigen. They are also referred to as near patient or point-of-care tests. These tests detect both influenza A and influenza B infections and may or may not distinguish between them. They vary in their complexity, the type of respiratory specimens acceptable for testing and the time needed to produce results. Rapid tests are useful for rapidly establishing the presence of influenza in certain circumstances such as outbreak situations, remote locations and areas where there is no access to laboratory facilities. However, WHO recommends that where possible tests such as IFA, culture or RT-PCR should be used to confirm and extend the results. Detailed WHO recommendations can be found at: www.who.int/csr/disease/avian_influenza/guidelines/rapid_testing/en/index.html

Materials required for IFA
Equipment

Fluorescence microscope	Centrifuge (low speed)
Incubator (optional)	

Supplies

Microscope slides (12 circles) Clay Adams – cat. no. 3032	Coverslips (24 mm x 60 mm) Corning – cat. no. 583331
Pipettes (1 ml) BD Biosciences (Falcon) – cat. no. 357503	Tissue culture (e.g. MDCK cells)
Glass beads (1–3 mm diameter)	Humid chamber
Centrifuge tubes (conical, 15ml) BD Biosciences (Falcon) – cat. no. 352097	Forceps or gloves

Buffers and reagents

Respiratory Panel Viral Screening and Identification Kit Chemicon International Inc – cat. no. 3105	Trypsin-EDTA (0.05% trypsin; 0.53 mM EDTA · 4Na) Invitrogen – cat. no. 25300-054
Acetone Fisher Scientific – cat. no. S93106	Water (distilled)

Preparation of solution and slides

The test is carried out following the instructions included in a commercial Respiratory Panel Viral Screening and Identification Kit. The quality of each slide prepared from a clinical specimen or isolate has to be evaluated by microscopy before the slide is fixed. Always use positive control slides and a negative control slide when testing.

Kit contents

- Antigen-positive control slides for influenza A and B; parainfluenza 1, 2 and 3; adenovirus; and respiratory syncytial virus.
- Monoclonal antibodies for influenza A and B; parainfluenza 1, 2 and 3; adenovirus; and respiratory syncytial virus.
- Respiratory virus screening antibody – a pool for all viruses listed above.
- Normal mouse antibody to be used as a negative control.
- Anti-mouse IgG:fluorescein isothiocyanate (IgG:FITC) conjugate.
- PBS salts.
- Tween 20/sodium azide solution (100x concentrate).
- Mounting fluid for slides.

Preparing PBS-Tween 20 solution (components in kit)

a. Dissolve the contents of the PBS packet in 950 ml of distilled water.
b. Add the Tween 20/sodium azide 100x concentrate (10 ml) to the PBS and mix.
c. Add 40 ml of distilled water to bring the total volume to 1 litre.

Preparing slides

1. After inoculation of the specimen and appropriate incubation for 3–4 days and/or observance of 1+ cytopathic effect (>25%), use a pipette to aspirate the medium from the tissue culture from each unknown specimen and from the cell control (uninoculated tissue culture to provide a negative control). Any extra medium from the infected cells may be frozen at -70 °C until testing has been completed. Positive control slides are included in the kit.
2. Rinse the cell monolayer gently 3 times with 1–2 ml PBS. Add 100 µl trypsin-EDTA and let it stand for 30 seconds. Gently tap the container to loosen cells.
3. Add 1 ml PBS. Centrifuge the cell suspension at 2000 rpm for 10 minutes in a conical tube. Resuspend the cell pellet in approximately 200 µl of PBS.
4. For each specimen, place 1 drop (15–20 µl) of cell suspension onto 9 circles on a single acetone-cleaned slide. On a separate slide, place 1 drop of cell suspension from the uninfected tissue culture onto 9 circles to serve as a negative control. Dry in an incubator or air dry at room temperature. The quality of each slide has to be evaluated by microscopy before the slide is fixed. Slides must exhibit at least 3 cells per field at 400x magnification to be considered adequate for detection.
5. Fix the slide in chilled acetone for 10 minutes and air dry completely. Slides may be stored for several months at -20 °C. ***Caution: acetone fixation does not necessarily eliminate the infectivity of either enveloped or non-enveloped viruses. Slides should therefore be considered infectious and handled appropriately (with forceps or gloves). Autoclave slides when the assay is finished.***

Staining procedure

1. Prepare the PBS-Tween 20 solution (see above) before starting the staining procedure.
2. Allow the slides from step **5** above to equilibrate to room temperature.
3. To three separate cell spots on each of the slides, add 1 drop of the virus-specific monoclonal antibodies, 1 drop of the respiratory virus screening antibody and 1 drop of the negative control normal mouse antibody.
4. Carefully place slides in a humid chamber and incubate at 37 °C for 30 minutes.
5. Rinse slides thoroughly but gently with PBS-Tween 20 solution for 10–15 seconds. At no step should the slides dry completely once the staining process has been started.
6. Shake off excess buffer.
7. Add sufficient anti-mouse IgG:FITC conjugate to each cell spot to cover the entire area on which cells have been deposited.
8. Carefully place slides in a humid chamber and incubate at 37 °C for 30 minutes.
9. Rinse slides thoroughly with PBS-Tween 20 solution.
10. Shake off excess buffer.
11. Add one drop of mounting fluid to the centre of the slide.
12. Carefully place a coverslip on the slide – avoid getting air bubbles trapped between the slide and coverslip.
13. View slides under a fluorescence microscope at 100–200x magnification to find cells that are fluorescing. Use 400x magnification for more detailed examination.

Interpretation of results

First check that there is an adequate cell density on the slide and then carefully view the entire area of the preparation. Any extracellular staining or cell fragments showing fluorescence should be regarded as nonspecific staining. One or more intact cells showing a specific staining pattern can be accepted as a positive result.

Specific staining should be of an intense apple-green appearance and must always be located intracellularly (**FIGURE 2.J-1A**). The pattern of staining is often granular, but larger inclusions may be homogeneously stained (**FIGURE 2.J-1B**). With the monoclonal antibodies against influenza viruses A and B, nuclear and/or cytoplasmic staining can be observed. Nuclear and/or cytoplasmic staining is also observed with the monoclonal antibody against adenovirus, while antibodies against respiratory syncytial virus and parainfluenza viruses give cytoplasmic staining. The mounting fluid contains Evans Blue which gives a dark-red appearance to uninfected cells.

FIGURE 2.J-1
Staining patterns of cells infected with influenza viruses showing fluorescein isothiocyanate staining of antigen-antibody complexes in cells[a]

A: Mink cells infected with influenza A

B: Primary monkey kidney cells infected with influenza B

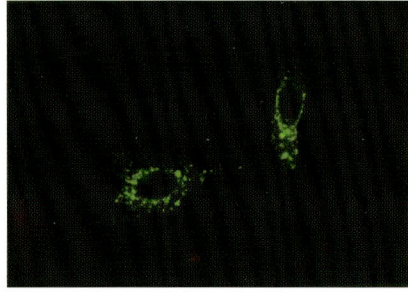
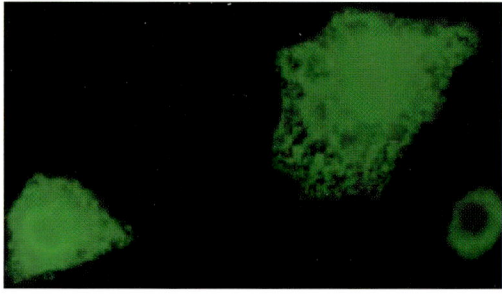

[a] Source: Chemicon now a part of Millipore.

Quality control

Control slides with infected and uninfected cells are included in each kit. These slides provide an appropriate control for the monoclonal antibodies and the conjugate. Viewing these slides will help the performer of the test to become familiar with the specific staining pattern of each monoclonal antibody. The quality of each slide prepared from a clinical specimen or isolate has to be evaluated by microscopy before the slide is fixed. In particular, there must be a sufficiently high number of epithelial cells on the preparation, and mucus must have been removed.

Limitations of IFA staining

As stated above, the quality of the clinical specimen is of the utmost importance for successful performance of the test. Virus-infected epithelial cells in a clinical specimen are very labile and may easily be damaged by inappropriate handling or by extended storage before processing. It is therefore mandatory that all specimens for IFA staining are placed on ice immediately after collection and kept cold until processed. Vigorous pipetting or pelleting cells at centrifugal forces exceeding 500x g may also damage infected cells.

The number of infected cells that may be obtained by washing, swabbing or aspiration decreases during the course of infection. It is therefore advisable that specimens are taken as soon as possible after the onset of symptoms, and preferably during the first 3 days of illness (see **SECTION 2.A**).

IFA staining of infected cells with monoclonal antibodies is also a highly specific method, and only viruses for which specific antibodies are available can be detected by this technique.

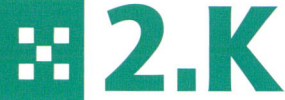

2.K
Use of neuraminidase inhibition assays to determine the susceptibility of influenza viruses to antiviral drugs

The two classes of licensed antiviral drugs available for the treatment and prophylaxis of influenza are the adamantanes and the neuraminidase (NA) inhibitors. Adamantanes target the proton channel formed by the M2 protein and are therefore only effective against influenza A viruses since influenza B viruses lack this protein. In 2006, following the rapid emergence of widespread resistance to this class of influenza antivirals, the United States Centers for Disease Control and Prevention (CDC) recommended that the adamantanes no longer be used in the treatment and prophylaxis of influenza virus infections. The two currently available NA inhibitors – zanamivir and oseltamivir – therefore became the only drugs recommended for the treatment and prophylaxis of both influenza A and B infections. Both these drugs (as well as the candidate drug peramivir) were developed to act specifically against viral NA which removes the terminal sialic acid present on cellular receptors (to which haemagglutinin binds) and on virus glycoproteins to promote the release of progeny virions from infected cells thus facilitating their dispersal in the respiratory tract. Early treatment with either drug reduces both the severity and duration of influenza symptoms and associated complications.

The emergence of marked resistance to oseltamivir among seasonal A(H1N1) viruses during late 2007 to early 2008 has made it imperative to conduct NA inhibitor susceptibility surveillance among circulating influenza viruses worldwide.

The following two approaches are described in this section:[1]

A. At the CDC in the United States, a chemiluminescent neuraminidase inhibition (NAI) assay is used as a primary tool to assess the susceptibility of current circulating seasonal influenza isolates to the NA inhibitors zanamivir and oseltamivir. The assay was chosen because it requires a small volume of virus, even for a low-titre virus preparation. The other advantage is that the reagents are provided in the form of a kit (NA-Star from Applied Biosystems). Although the kit includes a protocol supplied by the manufacturer, there are several differences between this protocol and the actual protocol used at the CDC as outlined below.

B. At the National Institute for Medical Research (NIMR) in the United Kingdom, NA activity and drug susceptibility are measured using the fluorescent substrate 2'-(4-methylumbelliferyl)-a-D-N-acetylneuraminic acid (MUNANA). This assay when

---

[1] It should be noted however that a range of other methods have also been developed for this purpose. For example, at the Health Protection Agency (HPA) of the United Kingdom a method for amplifying and pyrosequencing the (H1) N1 gene (from nucleotide 601 to 931) is used to detect the H275Y mutation which causes resistance to oseltamivir (see: Lackenby et al., 2008). Other mutations not detected by this method however can result in resistance.

performed in the presence of inhibitors allows the concentration of drug required to inhibit enzyme activity by 50% (IC_{50}) to be determined. The assay has been used to assess the susceptibility of circulating seasonal influenza; of sporadic zoonoses (such as H5N1 and H7N7); and of pandemic (H1N1) 2009 isolates.

Note: whichever method is used a local risk assessment should be conducted and a suitable level of biosafety containment used, especially for viruses with pandemic potential.

A. THE CDC CHEMILUMINESCENT NAI ASSAY

Materials required
NA-Star Kit

The NA-Star Kit is a complete kit containing the following required reagents and plates and is obtained from **Applied Biosystems (cat. no. 4374422)**:

NA-Star assay buffer **Applied Biosystems – cat. no. 4374345**
NA-Star substrate buffer **Applied Biosystems – cat. no. 4374347**
NA-Star accelerator **Applied Biosystems – cat. no. 4374346**
Opaque 96-well white plates **Applied Biosystems – cat. no. 4374349**
NA-Star reagent **Applied Biosystems – cat. no. 4374348**

Zanamivir **GlaxoSmithKline**
Oseltamivir – the active metabolite of the prodrug oseltamivir (oseltamivir carboxylate) ***must*** be used and is provided to CDC by **Hoffman-La Roche**.
Reference virus strains – virus stocks must be stored at -70 °C. Do not use freeze-thawed reference viruses. Take a fresh aliquot of the reference viruses (sensitive and resistant controls) to be used for each assay.

Equipment

Fridge (4 °C) (for storage of drug dilutions)	Freezers (-20 °C for drug stock storage; and -70 °C for long-term virus storage)
96-well plate reader for luminescence with injector	Software for curve fitting and IC50 calculations
Incubator (37 °C)	

Supplies

Reagent reservoirs for NA-Star buffer and NA inhibitor dilutions	15 ml and 50 ml conical tubes for substrate and accelerator solutions
1.5 ml tubes for virus dilutions	Assorted sizes of pipettes and pipette tips, plus pipetting device
Multichannel pipetter **Rainin – cat. no. L12-200**	Tips for multichannel pipetter **Rainin – cat. no. RT-L200F**

Chemiluminescent neuraminidase inhibition (NAI) assay procedure
Step 1: Neuraminidase (NA) activity assay to determine working virus dilution

Multiple aliquots of all control viruses should be pre-prepared and stored at -70 oC. Prior to performing the NA activity assay:

a. thaw the control viruses to be used in a class-II biosafety cabinet;
b. thaw the virus isolates to be assayed in a class-II biosafety cabinet;
c. bring all reagents to room temperature; and
d. turn on plate reader to be used, and prime the injector to be used with NA-Star accelerator reagent.

For the NA activity assay, a total of 16 viruses may be assayed on a single 96-well plate (see **FIGURE 2.K-1** below). The use of both drug-sensitive and drug-resistant control viruses of the appropriate influenza subtype allows for an assessment to be made of the drug susceptibilities of the virus isolates being tested. For each influenza subtype to be tested, a matching pair of reference viruses (one sensitive (S) and one resistant (R) to the NA inhibitor compounds oseltamivir and/or zanamivir) should be used in each assay run. **TABLE 2.K-1** presents an example of the paired drug-sensitive and drug-resistant reference viruses used by CDC for each NA subtype.

TABLE 2.K-1
Example of drug-sensitive and drug-resistant control virus pairs used at CDC

Subtype	Reference virus	Mutation
H1N1 (oseltamivir)	A/Georgia/17/2006 (S) A/Georgia/20/2006 (R)	Wild type H274Y (N2 numbering)
H3N2 (oseltamivir)	A/Washington/01/2007 (S) A/Texas/12/2007 (R)	Wild type E119V (N2 numbering)
Influenza B (zanamivir and oseltamivir)	B/Memphis/20/96 (S) B/Memphis/20/96 (R)	Wild type R152K (N2 numbering)

To perform the NA activity assay, 2-fold serial dilutions of each virus are assayed in a 96-well plate in the presence of the NA-Star substrate buffer. The measurement of the NA activity of each virus prior to the NAI assay is useful in ensuring that the data obtained are reproducible and reliable. To ensure NAI assay integrity it has been shown that the optimal ratio of NA activity (signal) to background noise is between 10:1 and 40:1. The NA activity assay enables determination of the amount of virus needed in the NAI assay to achieve the required ratio. Too low a level of NA activity will result in false drug resistance being observed while too high an activity level will result in non-reproducible data.

1. Add 80 μl of NA-Star assay buffer to all wells in columns 1 and 7 of a 96-well plate, and then add 50 μl NA-Star assay buffer to all the wells of columns 2–5 and 8–11.
2. Add 50 μl NA-Star assay buffer to all the wells of columns 6 and 12 as a blank control.
3. In a class-II biosafety cabinet prepare an initial 1:5 dilution of the first 8 viruses to be assayed by adding 20 μl of each virus to be tested to the corresponding well in column 1 of each row – i.e. one row per virus.

4. Using a multichannel pipetter, perform serial 2-fold dilutions of the first 8 viruses to be tested in rows A–H by pipetting up and down three times in column 1 and then removing 50 μl from the well and adding it to the next well. Do this for columns 2–5, discarding the last 50 μl from column 5 to leave column 6 as a blank control.
5. Repeat as above with the next batch of 8 viruses to be tested in columns 7–11. As with column 6, column 12 is kept as a blank control by discarding the 50 μl removed from column 11.
6. A graphic summary of the above sequences is shown in **FIGURE 2.K-1**.
7. For each assay, prepare a fresh working stock dilution of NA-Star substrate buffer. A 1:1000 dilution of NA-Star substrate buffer in NA-Star assay buffer is required both for the NA activity assay and the NAI assay (e.g. 20 μl NA-Star substrate buffer in 20 ml NA-Star assay buffer).
8. Using a multichannel repeater pipette, add 10 μl of the working stock dilution of NA-Star substrate buffer to each of the 6 columns for each virus being tested, starting with column 6 back to column 1 for the first 8 viruses on the plate. Ensure that the pipette tips are positioned in the bottom of each well to guarantee correct dispensation of the substrate.
9. Change pipette tips and repeat for the next batch of 8 viruses in rows 1–8, columns 12–7. After addition of the NA-Star substrate buffer, tap the plate gently on each side to mix the virus and NA-Star substrate buffer.
10. Allow the plates to stand at room temperature for 30 minutes.
11. To measure NA activity, place the 96-well plate in the luminescence plate reader and start the relevant programme to be used. The programme will need to dispense 60 μl of NA-Star accelerator to each well of the plate and to then measure the readout of each well after a 1 second delay following the addition of accelerator.

FIGURE 2.K-1
Virus 2-fold serial dilutions

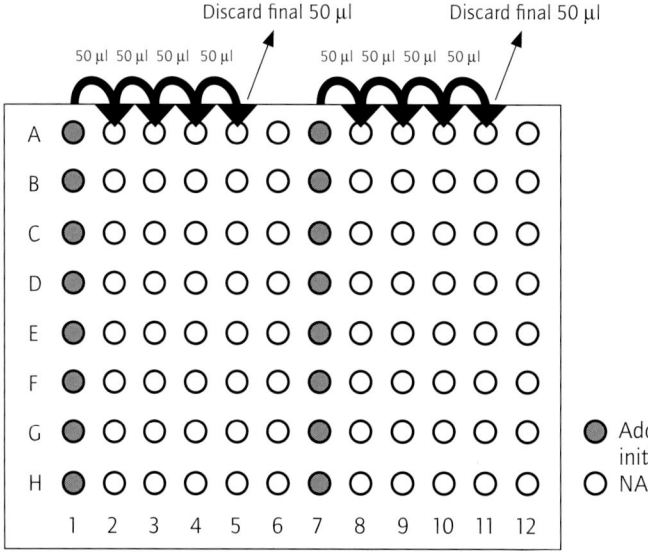

As previously mentioned, the virus dilution that gives a <40 and >10 signal-to-noise ratio is considered to be the optimal virus dilution for use in the NAI assay.

Note: virus isolates must be diluted at least 1:5 with NA-Star assay buffer to reduce the signal-quenching effect of the phenol red present in tissue culture media.

Step 2: NAI assay for the determination of IC_{50} value

Up to 8 viruses may be assayed for NAI on a single 96-well plate, one row per virus to be tested across columns 1–11. Again, the inclusion of a pair of drug-sensitive and drug-resistant viruses for each NA subtype to be tested in each assay run is strongly recommended.

Optimal dilutions of each virus isolate (calculated from the data obtained in the NA activity assay above) should be assayed on 2 separate 96-well plates in the presence of NA-Star substrate buffer. On one plate the susceptibility of virus isolates to the NA inhibitor zanamivir is measured, and on the second plate their susceptibility to the NA inhibitor oseltamivir is measured.

1. In a class-II biosafety cabinet take a 1.5 ml tube and prepare 800 µl of the working dilution for each virus to be assayed (as determined in step 1 above) using NA-Star assay buffer. This will ensure a sufficient volume of diluted virus to test against the two NA inhibitors.
2. Using the 50 µM stock of each drug, prepare the required half-log10 dilutions of both zanamivir and oseltamivir in NA-Star assay buffer in accordance with **TABLE 2.K-2**.
3. To each well in column 12 of both 96-well assay plates add 50 µl NA-Star assay buffer as a blank control. To the wells in column 11 add 25 µl of NA-Star assay buffer. This will act as another control as it will contain the respective virus and NA-Star substrate buffer in the absence of any drug.
4. To all other wells on each of the plates add 25 µl of the corresponding drug dilution, with the lowest drug concentration in column 10 through to the highest drug concentration in column 1. If the drug solution is added starting from the wells in column 10 back to the wells in column 1, the same pipette tip can be used for the entire plate used for each respective drug.
5. Using a multichannel pipette, add 25 µl of each virus dilution to columns 1–11 of the relevant row for that virus. Start at column 11 and add towards column 1 – i.e. from the lowest drug dilution to the highest drug dilution. Following addition of the virus, tap the plates gently on each side to mix the virus and drug solutions.
6. Incubate the plates at 37 °C for 30 minutes. If a 37 °C incubator is not available, the plates can be allowed to stand at room temperature for 30 minutes.
7. Following incubation, add 10 µl of NA-Star substrate buffer to the bottom of each well using a multichannel pipette. Remember to start from the lowest drug concentration through to the highest concentration (i.e. from column 12 through to column 1). Following addition of the NA-Star substrate buffer, tap the plates gently on each side to mix the buffer, virus and drug solutions.[1]

---

[1] It is important to stagger the addition of NA-Star substrate buffer if multiple plates are used to account for the time it takes to read each plate using the plate reader. For the approach currently used at CDC it takes approximately 7 minutes for each plate to be read. The addition of NA-Star substrate buffer to each subsequent plate is therefore staggered by 7 minutes.

8. Allow the plates to stand at room temperature for 30 minutes.
9. Place the 96-well plate in the luminescence plate reader and start the relevant programme to be used. The programme will need to dispense 60 µl of NA-Star accelerator to each well of the plate and to measure the readout of each well after a 1-second delay following addition of the accelerator.
10. After reading the plate, export the data as either a text or Excel file depending upon the requirements of the validated software used for the calculation of the IC_{50} values. The IC_{50} value is the concentration of a drug required to inhibit enzymatic activity by 50%.
11. Curve fitting and IC_{50} values are determined by the equation:
   $y = V_{max} \{1-[x/(K + x)]\}$ – where y is the enzyme activity being inhibited; V_{max} is the maximum reaction rate (using in-house CDC *JASPR* software or in-house GlaxoSmithKline *Robosage* software); x is the inhibitor concentration; and K is the IC50 for the inhibition curve (that is, y = 50% V_{max} when x = K). Enzyme activity is measured as relative light units (RLU).

For further information on IC_{50} data interpretation, please refer to Okomo-Adhiambo et al. (2010); Sheu et al. (2008); and Wetherall et al. (2003).

TABLE 2.K-2
Neuraminidase inhibitor half-log10 dilutions

Inhibitor dilution #	Volumes of NA inhibitor and NA-Star assay buffer required for each dilution	Required approximate conc (nM)	Final approximate conc (nM)[a]
1	30 µl of 50 µM stock of inhibitor + 720 µl NA-Star assay buffer	2000	1000
2	250 µl of dilution 1 + 540 µl NA-Star assay buffer	633	316
3	250 µl of dilution 2 + 540 µl NA-Star assay buffer	200	100
4	250 µl of dilution 3 + 540 µl NA-Star assay buffer	63.4	31.7
5	250 µl of dilution 4 + 540 µl NA-Star assay buffer	20	10
6	250 µl of dilution 5 + 540 µl NA-Star assay buffer	6.3	3.18
7	250 µl of dilution 6 + 540 µl NA-Star assay buffer	2	1.01
8	250 µl of dilution 7 + 540 µl NA-Star assay buffer	0.64	0.32
9	250 µl of dilution 8 + 540 µl NA-Star assay buffer	0.20	0.10
10	250 µl of dilution 9 + 540 µl NA-Star assay buffer	0.06	0.032

[a] The final concentration does not account for 10 µl of NA-Star substrate buffer.

A number of possible causes of potential problems associated with the interpretation of the chemiluminescent NAI assay, along with their recommended solutions, are shown in **TABLE 2.K-3**.

TABLE 2.K-3
Possible causes of problems associated with the interpretation of the chemiluminescent NAI assay, and their recommended solutions

Problem	Possible cause(s)	Solution
Weak or no NA activity/signal	i) Problem with the virus dilution used	i) Re-check NA activity data and calculation of virus dilution to be used
	ii) Too little NA-Star substrate buffer added	ii) Re-run the assay ensuring correct addition of substrate to the bottom of each well
	iii) Reagents too cold for the chemistry to be accurately executed	iii) Repeat with reagents which have been allowed to warm to room temperature
	iv) Insufficient incubation	iv) Repeat assay ensuring correct incubation times are adhered to
	v) NA content in virus preparation too low	v) Re-grow virus
	vi) Accelerator not added to reaction	vi) Check accelerator volume in machine
Uncharacteristically high IC_{50} value	i) Too little virus added to assay	i) Repeat the assay with more virus
	ii) Possible contamination of influenza A with an influenza B virus	ii) Check sample by running real-time RT-PCR analysis to check for co-infection with an influenza B virus
	iii) Incorrect concentration of drug present at each dilution	iii) Repeat the assay using fresh drug dilutions
	iv) Possible mixed infection with another pathogen which exhibits NA acticity (e.g. paramyxovirus)	iv) Perform RT-PCR with paramyxovirus-specific primers

Where facilities exist, conventional sequencing or pyrosequencing can be performed on the NA gene to check for the presence of molecular markers of resistance.

B. THE NIMR MUNANA NAI ASSAY

The procedure presented below has been based upon the NIMR MUNANA approach and is suitable for use with clinical isolates, tissue culture and egg-grown influenza A and B viruses.

Materials required
Equipment

96-well fluorescence plate reader **Biotek – Synergy 2 Multi-Mode Microplate Reader**	Incubator (37 °C)
Fridge (4 °C)	Freezers (-20 °C and -80 °C)
Laboratory shaker	

Supplies

Black 96-well microtitre plates (flat bottom) **Corning – cat. no. 3915**	Reagent reservoirs for substrate/stop solution **Fisher Scientific – cat. no. PMP-331-010C**
8-well and 12-well multichannel pipettes **Thermo Scientific – cat. nos. 4661010 & 4661070**	Pipette tips for multichannel pipettes

Reagents

2-morpholinoethenesulfonic acid (MES) Sigma-Aldrich – cat. no. M3885	Calcium chloride Fisher Scientific – cat. no. C/1280NC/53
Oseltamivir carboxylate Roche – cat. no. GS4071	Zanamivir Glaxo-Smithkline – cat. no. GR121167X or GG167
2'-(4-methylumbelliferyl)-a-D-N-acetyl neuraminic acid (MUNANA) Sigma-Aldrich – cat. no. M8639	Glycine Fisher Scientific – cat. no. BPE381-5
Ethanol absolute Fisher Scientific – cat. no. E/0665/15	Sodium hydroxide Fisher Scientific – cat. no. BPE359-212

Cells, buffers and other materials

100 µM oseltamivir carboxylate (3.5 µM stock solution in H_2O)	100 µM zanamivir (3.5 µM stock solution in H_2O)
MES buffer (32.5 µM MES, 4 mM $CaCl_2$, pH 6.5)	100 µM MUNANA (1 mM stock in MES buffer)
Stop solution (0.1 M glycine, 25% ethanol, pH 10.7)	

MUNANA neuraminidase inhibition (NAI) assay procedure
Step 1: Neuraminidase (NA) activity assay to determine working virus dilution

For the NA activity assay, a total of four viruses may be assayed on a single 96-well microtitre plate. For each influenza subtype to be tested, a matching pair of reference viruses (one sensitive (S) and one resistant (R) to the NA inhibitor compounds oseltamivir and/or zanamivir) should be used in each assay run. **TABLE 2.K-4** presents an example of the paired drug-sensitive and drug-resistant reference viruses used by NIMR for each NA subtype.

TABLE 2.K-4
Example of drug-sensitive and drug-resistant control virus pairs used at NIMR

Subtype	Reference virus	Mutation
H1N1	A/Norway/1758/07 (S) A/Norway/1735/07 (R)	Wild type H275Y
H3N2 (oseltamivir)	A/Texas/1/77 (S) A/Texas/1/77 (R)	Wild type E119V
H3N2 (zanamivir)	A/Thuringen/76/08 (S) A/Thuringen/75/08 (R)	Wild type Q136K
Influenza B	B/Memphis/20/96 (S) B/Memphis/20/96 (R)	Wild type R152K

The enzymatic activity of each virus is measured using the fluorescent MUNANA substrate. This will enable the determination of the optimal virus sample dilution to be used to standardize virus NA activity when measuring IC_{50} values for the NA inhibitors. As described below, each virus sample is initially titrated by making serial 2-fold dilutions in a black 96-well microtitre plate and is then assayed in the presence of MUNANA. The optimal virus sample dilutions fall in the linear portion of the enzyme activity curve and are determined graphically as shown in **FIGURE 2.K-2**.

FIGURE 2.K-2
Neuraminidase enzyme activity curve – the horizontal line crosses in the linear portion of the enzyme activity curves

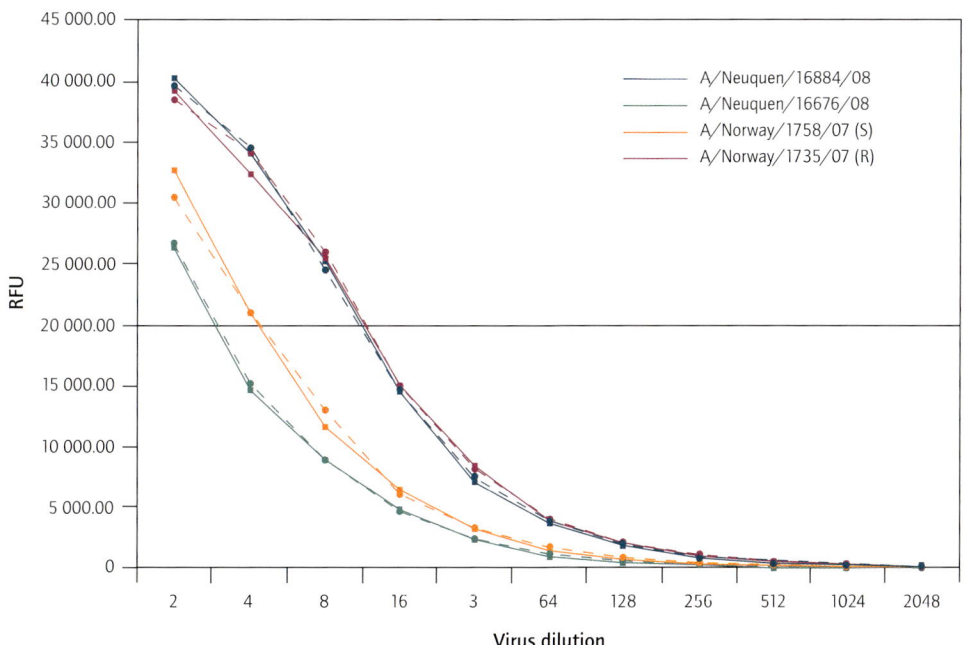

1. Add 20 µl MES buffer to each well.
2. Prepare duplicate 2-fold dilutions of each test virus as shown in **TABLE 2.K-5** (i.e. add 20 µl of the first virus to wells A1 and B1 giving a 1/2 dilution, mix virus and buffer several times, and then serially dilute along the plate as far as row 11 discarding the last 20 µl from row 11. Row 12 should contain 20 µl of MES buffer only.
3. Repeat for all other virus pairs down the plate (C1–11/D1–11 then E1–11/F1–11 etc.).
4. Prepare the MUNANA substrate at a concentration of 100 µM in MES buffer, and add 30 µl of substrate to each well – including the blanks in row 12.
5. Ensure the components of each well are mixed thoroughly by shaking for up to 30 seconds on a laboratory shaker at 200–300 rpm. Cover or seal plate and incubate at 37 °C for 60 minutes.
6. Terminate the reaction by adding 150 µl of stop solution to each well.
7. Place the plate(s) in the fluorimeter, and detect fluorescence at an excitation wavelength of 355 nm and emission at 460 nm.
8. The average of the blank-only wells should then be subtracted from all other data points and the resulting values plotted as Relative Fluorescence Units (RFU) against virus dilution.
9. The optimal virus sample dilution can then be determined graphically from the linear portion of the enzyme activity curve (**FIGURE 2.K-2**).

TABLE 2.K-5
Plate layout for the determination of optimal virus dilution

Virus dilution		1/2	1/4	1/8	1/16	1/32	1/64	1/128	1/256	1/512	1/1024	1/2048	Buff
	wells	1	2	3	4	5	6	7	8	9	10	11	12
Virus 1	A										→		
Virus 1	B										→		
Virus 2	C										→		
Virus 2	D										→		
Virus 3	E										→		
Virus 3	F										→		
Virus 4	G										→		
Virus 4	H										→		

Step 2: NAI assay for the determination of IC_{50} value

Up to 4 viruses (in duplicate) can be assayed for NAI on a single 96-well microtitre plate (**TABLE 2.K-6**). Each assay run should include paired drug-sensitive and drug-resistant viruses for each NA subtype being tested. The optimal dilution of each virus (as determined above in the MUNANA assay) should be assayed on two separate 96-well microtitre plates. This will enable the susceptibility of each of the viruses to oseltamivir and zanamivir to be measured simultaneously.

Ideally IC_{50} determination should be performed on the same day as the activity assay. If this is not possible then no more than 24 hours should elapse between assays. **Note: only samples with HA titres of 16 and over can be reliably tested to give accurate IC_{50} values. This is due to samples with low HA titre possibly not having sufficient NA activity for inhibition testing. Samples with low HA titre should be passaged to yield higher titres.**

Viruses should be stored at 4 °C at all times between assays. This is due to possible instability of the NA activity of resistant viruses carrying mutations either in – or in close proximity to – their active site. **Note: virus isolates stored at -80 °C can be thawed and their IC_{50} analysed. After thawing, store at 4 °C until IC_{50} testing is complete.**

TABLE 2.K-6
Plate layout for virus addition during NAI assay

		1	2	3	4	5	6	7	8	9	10	11	12
Virus 1	A										→		
Virus 1	B										→		
Virus 2	C										→		
Virus 2	D										→		
Virus 3	E										→		
Virus 3	F										→		
Virus 4	G										→		
Virus 4	H										→		

TABLE 2.K-7
Drug dilution preparation

Step[a]	Dilution series	Drug Concentration (nM)	"In assay" Concentration (nM)
1	400 µl of 100 µM working stock+1600 µl MES	20 000	4000
2	600 µl of step 1 +1800 µl MES	5000	1000
3	600 µl of step 2 +1800 µl MES	1250	250
4	600 µl of step 3 +1800 µl MES	312.5	62.5
5	600 µl of step 4 +1800 µl MES	78.13	15.63
6	600 µl of step 5 +1800 µl MES	19.53	3.91
7	600 µl of step 6 +1800 µl MES	4.88	0.98
8	600 µl of step 7 +1800 µl MES	1.22	0.24
9	600 µl of step 8 +1800 µl MES	0.31	0.061
10	600 µl of step 9 +1800 µl MES	0.076	0.015
11	Buffer only	Virus/Substrate control	0
12	Buffer only	Substrate/Buffer control	0

[a] Steps 1-12 correspond to the plate column numbers as shown in **TABLE 2.K-6**.

1. Optimally dilute each virus in MES assay buffer in accordance with the results of the NA activity assay.
2. Add 10 µl of diluted test virus 1 to the first 2 rows (A+B) of wells 1–11 and so on for the other test viruses.
3. Add 10 µl of MES buffer to all rows (A–H) of column 12.
4. Prepare 4-fold dilutions of drug(s) starting at 20 µM (**TABLE 2.K-7**).
5. Add 10 µl of each drug dilution to a complete column of the 96-well microtitre plate (i.e. column 1 (A–H): 20 000 nM; column 2 (A–H): 2000 nM etc. as far as column 10. Add 10 µl of MES buffer to columns 11 and 12.
6. Ensure the components of each well are mixed thoroughly by shaking for up to 30 seconds on a laboratory shaker at 200–300 rpm. Cover or seal the plate and incubate at 37 °C for 30 minutes.
7. Prepare 3 ml of the MUNANA working stock (100 µM) for each 96-well microtitre plate, and add 30 µl of the substrate to each well.
8. Ensure the components of each well are mixed thoroughly by shaking for up to 30 seconds on a laboratory shaker at 200–300 rpm. Cover or seal the plate and incubate at 37 °C for 60 minutes.
9. The reaction is terminated by the addition of 150 µl of stop solution to all wells.
10. Place the plate(s) in the fluorimeter, and detect fluorescence using an excitation wavelength of 355 nm and an emission wavelength of 460 nm.
11. The average of the blank-only wells should once again be subtracted from all data points. The data can then be plotted as Relative Fluorescence Units (RFU) against NA inhibitor concentration. This should yield a sigmoid dose-response curve as shown in **FIGURE 2.K-3**.
12. Data-analysis software incorporating an IC_{50} function (such as *GraFit 6.0*) can be used for curve fitting and for the accurate calculation of IC_{50} values. After reading

FIGURE 2.K-3
Sigmoid dose response curve of neuraminidase inhibition

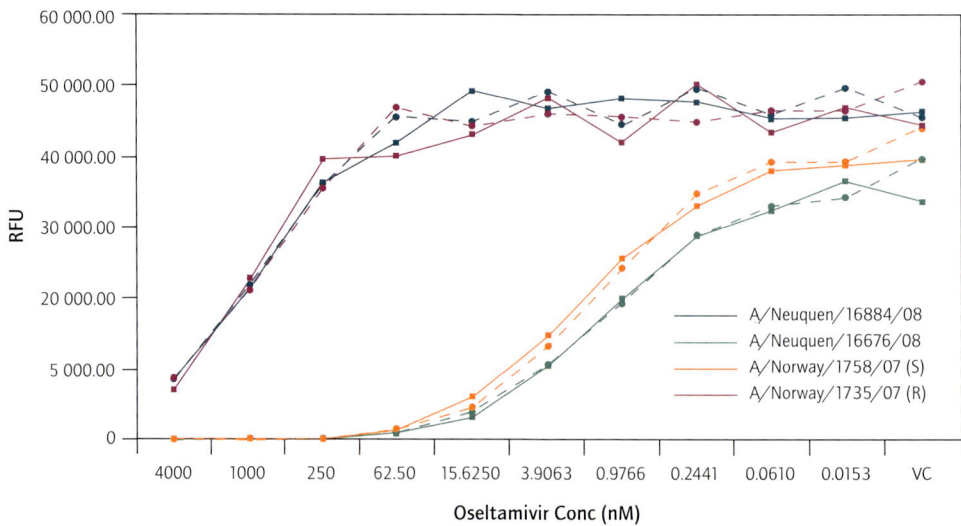

the plate(s) export the data as either a text file or an Excel file depending upon the requirements of the validated software to be used.

Where facilities exist, conventional sequencing or pyrosequencing can be performed on the NA gene to check for the presence of molecular markers of resistance. **TABLE 2.K-8** shows the drug susceptibilities of a range of known NA mutations.

TABLE 2.K-8
Drug susceptibility of influenza A and B viruses

Virus type/subtype	NA mutation	Drug susceptibility[a]		
		oseltamivir	zanamivir	peramivir
(A)H3N2	R292K	R	"R"	R
	E119V	R	S	S
	E119V + I222V	R	S	"R"
	N294S	"R"	S	S
	Δ244-247	R	S	
	Q136K	S	R	
(A)H1N1	H275Y	R	S	R
	Q136K	S	R	
(A)H5N1	H275Y	R	S	
	N295S	"R"	S	
(B)	D198N	"R"	"R"	S
	R152K	R	R	R

[a] Determined by NA assay.
R = high level resistance.
"R" = intermediate reduction in drug susceptibility.
S = sensitive.

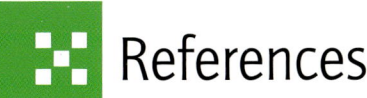
References

Arden A et al. (1995). Vaccine Use and the Risk of Outbreaks in a Sample of Nursing Homes during an Influenza. *American Journal of Public Health*, 85(3):399–401.

Aymard-Henry MT et al. (1973). Influenza virus neuraminidase and neuraminidase inhibition test procedures. *Bulletin of the World Health Organization*, 48:199–202.

Barker WH, Mullooly JP (1982). Pneumonia and influenza deaths during epidemics: implications for prevention. *Archives of Internal Medicine*, 142(1):85–89.

Brotherton JML et al. (2003). A large outbreak of influenza A and B on a cruise ship causing widespread morbidity. *Epidemiology and Infection*, 130(2003):263–271.

Burch J et al. (2009). Prescription of anti-influenza drugs for healthy adults: a systematic review and meta-analysis. *The Lancet Infectious Diseases*, 9(9):537–545.

Freshney RI (2005). *Culture of animal cells: a manual of basic technique* (5th ed.). Hoboken, NJ, Wiley-Liss.

Hartert TV et al. (2003). Maternal morbidity and perinatal outcomes among pregnant women with respiratory hospitalizations during influenza season. *American Journal of Obstetrics & Gynecology*, 189(6):1705–1712.

Hirst GK (1942). The quantitative determination of influenza virus and antibodies by means of red cell agglutination. *The Journal of Experimental Medicine*, 75:47–64.

Izurieta HS et al. (2000). Influenza and the rates of hospitalization for respiratory disease among infants and young children. *New England Journal of Medicine*, 342(23):1752–1753.

Kärber G (1931). 50% end-point calculation. *Archiv für Experimentelle Pathologie und Pharmakologie*, 162:480–483.

Lackenby A et al. (2008). Rapid quantitation of neuraminidase inhibitor drug resistance in influenza virus quasispecies. *Antiviral Therapy*, 13(6):809–820.

Lipatov AS et al. (2004). Influenza: emergence and control. *Journal of Virology*, 78:8951–8959.

Lyytikäinen O et al. (1998). Influenza A outbreak among adolescents in a ski hostel. *European Journal of Clinical Microbiology & Infectious Diseases*, 17(2):128–130.

Okomo-Adhiambo M et al. (2010). Neuraminidase Inhibitor Susceptibility Testing in Human Influenza Viruses: A Laboratory Surveillance Perspective. *Viruses – Antivirals Against Influenza* (Special Issue). Submitted.

Palese P (2004). Influenza: old and new threats. *Nature Medicine*, 10(Suppl. 12):S82–S87.

Reed LJ, Muench H (1938). A simple method of estimating fifty per cent endpoints. *American Journal of Hygiene*, 27:493–497.

Sheu TG et al. (2008). Surveillance for Neuraminidase Inhibitor Resistance among Human Influenza A and B Viruses Circulating Worldwide from 2004 to 2008. *Antimicrobial Agents and Chemotherapy*, 52(9):3284–3292.

Simonsen L et al. (2000). The impact of influenza epidemics on hospitalizations. *Journal of Infectious Diseases*, 181:831–837.

Smith NM et al. (2006). Prevention and control of influenza: recommendations of the Advisory Committee on Immunization Practices (ACIP). *Morbidity and Mortality Weekly Report*, 55:1–42. Erratum, *Morbidity and Mortality Weekly Report*, 2006, 55:800.

Thompson WW et al. (2003) Mortality associated with influenza and respiratory syncytial virus in the United States. *Journal of the American Association*, 289:179–186.

Thompson WW et al. (2004). Influenza-associated hospitalizations in the United States. *Journal of the American Association*, 292:1333–1340.

Warren L (1959). The thiobarbituric acid assay of sialic acids. *Journal of Biological Chemistry*, 234:1971–1975.

Wetherall NT et al. (2003). Evaluation of Neuraminidase Enzyme Assays Using Different Substrates to Measure Susceptibility of Influenza Virus Clinical Isolates to Neuraminidase Inhibitors: Report of the Neuraminidase Inhibitor Susceptibility Network. *Journal of Clinical Microbiology*, 41:742–750.

Wiedbrauk DL, Johnston SLG (1993). *Manual of Clinical Virology*. Raven Press, New York.

Zucs P et al. (2005). Influenza associated excess mortality in Germany, 1985–2001. *Emerging Themes in Epidemiology*, 2:6.

Bibliography

Influenza surveillance

Barr IG et al. (2010). Epidemiological, antigenic and genetic characteristics of seasonal influenza A(H1N1), A(H3N2) and B influenza viruses: basis for the WHO recommendation on the composition of influenza vaccines for use in the 2009–2010 Northern Hemisphere season. *Vaccine*, 28:1156–1167.

Brammer TL et al. (2002). Surveillance for influenza – United States, 1997–98, 1998–99, and 1999–00 seasons. MMWR Surveillance Summaries, Centers for Disease Control and Prevention. *Morbidity and Mortality Weekly Report*, 51(SS-7):1–10.

Dawood FS et al. (2009). Emergence of a Novel Swine-Origin Influenza A (H1N1) Virus in Humans: Novel Swine-Origin Influenza A (H1N1) Virus Investigation Team. *New England Journal of Medicine*, 360(25):2605–2615.

Gensheimer KF et al. (2002). Preparing for pandemic influenza: the need for enhanced surveillance. *Vaccine*, 20:S63–S65.

Glezen WP (1996). Emerging infections: pandemic influenza. *Epidemiologic Reviews*, 18:64–76.

Harper S et al. (2002). Influenza. Clinics in Laboratory Medicine, 22(4):863–882.

Klimov A et al. (1999). Surveillance and impact of influenza in the United States. *Vaccine*, 17(Suppl. 1):S42–S46.

Liu K-J, Kendal A (1987). Impact of influenza epidemics on mortality in the United States from October 1972 to May 1985. *American Journal of Public Health*, 77:712–716.

Noble GR (1982). Epidemiological and clinical aspects of influenza. In: Beare AS, ed. *Basic and applied influenza research*. Boca Raton, FL, CRC Press, 11–50.

Outbreak of swine-origin influenza A (H1N1) virus infection, Mexico, March–April 2009. Centers for Disease Control and Prevention. *Morbidity and Mortality Weekly Report*, 58(17):467–470.

Shaw MW et al. (2002). Reappearance and global spread of variants of influenza B/Victoria/2/87 lineage viruses in the 2000–2001 and 2001–2002 seasons. *Virology*, 303:1–8.

Simonsen L (1999). The global impact of influenza on morbidity and mortality. *Vaccine*, 17(Suppl. 1):S3–S10.

Taubenberger JK, Morens DM (2006). 1918 Influenza: the Mother of All Pandemics. *Emerging Infectious Diseases*, 12(1):15–22.

Thompson WW et al. (2003). Mortality associated with influenza and respiratory syncytial virus in the United States. *Journal of the American Medical Association*, 289:179–186.

Thompson WW et al. (2009). Estimates of US influenza-associated deaths made using four different methods. *Influenza & Other Respiratory Viruses*, 3(1):37–49.

Xu X et al. (2002). Intercontinental circulation of human influenza A(H1N2) reassortant viruses during the 2001/2002 influenza season. *The Journal of Infectious Diseases*, 186:1490–1493.

Ziegler T, Cox NJ (1995). Influenza viruses. In: Murray PR et al., eds. *Manual of clinical microbiology* (6th ed.). Washington, DC, American Society for Microbiology Press, 918–925.

Influenza control

Antigenic and genetic characteristics of influenza A(H5N1) and influenza A(H9N2) viruses and candidate vaccine viruses developed for potential use in human vaccines – February 2010. *Weekly Epidemiological Record*, 11(85):100–108.

Bridges CB et al. (2000). Effectiveness and cost-benefit of influenza vaccination of healthy working adults: A randomized controlled trial. *Journal of the American Medical Association*, 284:1655–1663.

Colman PM (2002). Neuraminidase inhibitors as antivirals. *Vaccine*, 20(Suppl. 2):S55–S58.

Couch RB (2000). Prevention and treatment of influenza. *New England Journal of Medicine*, 343:1778–1787.

Fiore AE et al. (2009). Prevention and control of seasonal influenza with vaccines. Recommendations of the Advisory Committee on Immunization Practices (ACIP), 2009. Recommendations and Reports, Centers for Disease Control and Prevention. *Morbidity and Mortality Weekly Report*, 58(RR-8):1–52.

Hayden FG (1997). Antivirals for pandemic influenza. *The Journal of Infectious Diseases*, 176(Suppl. 1):S56–S61.

Hayden FG. (2001). Perspectives on antiviral use during pandemic influenza. Philosophical Transactions of the Royal Society of London, Series B. *Biological Sciences*, 356:1877–1884.

Rudenko LG. (2000). Immunogenicity and efficacy of Russian live attenuated and U.S. inactivated influenza vaccines used alone and in combination in nursing home residents. *Vaccine*, 19:308–318.

Rudenko LG et al. (1996). Clinical and epidemiological evaluation of a live, cold-adapted influenza vaccine for 3–14-year-olds. *Bulletin of the World Health Organization*, 74:77–84.

Treanor J et al. (2002). Evaluation of a single dose of half strength inactivated influenza vaccine in healthy adults. *Vaccine*, 20:1099–1105.

Zambon M, Hayden FG (2001). Position statement: global neuraminidase inhibitor susceptibility network. *Antiviral Research*, 49:147–156.

Biosafety

Biosafety in Microbiological and Biomedical Laboratories at:
http://www.cdc.gov/biosafety/publications/bmbl5/index.htm

WHO Laboratory Biosafety Manual 3rd edition:
http://www.who.int/csr/resources/publications/biosafety/Biosafety7.pdf

WHO laboratory biosafety guidelines for handling specimens suspected of containing avian influenza A virus:
http://www.who.int/csr/disease/avian_influenza/guidelines/handlingspecimens/en/print.html

Collection and transport of clinical specimens

Johnson FB (1990). Transport of viral specimens. *Clinical Microbiology Reviews*, 3:120–131.

Lennette DE (1995). Collection and preparation of specimens for virological examination. In: Murray PR et al., eds. *Manual of clinical microbiology* (6th ed.). Washington, DC, American Society for Microbiology Press, 868–875.
www.who.int/csr/resources/publications/swineflu/storage_transport/en/index.html

Detection of influenza virus and antibodies

Chambers TM et al. (1994). Rapid diagnosis of equine influenza by the Directigen FLU-A enzyme immunoassay. *The Veterinary Record*, 135:275–279.

Espy MJ et al. (1986). Rapid detection of influenza viruses by shell vial assay with monoclonal antibodies. *Journal of Clinical Microbiology*, 24:677–679.

Gregory V et al. (2001). Infection of a child in Hong Kong by an influenza A H3N2 virus closely related to viruses circulating in European pigs. *Journal of General Virology*, 82:1397–1406.

Hancock K et al. (2009). Cross-Reactive Antibody Responses to the 2009 Pandemic H1N1 Influenza Virus. *New England Journal of Medicine*, 361:1945–1952.

McQuillin J, Madeley CR, Kendal AP (1985). Monoclonal antibodies for the rapid diagnosis of influenza A and B virus infections by immunofluorescence. *Lancet*, 2(8961):911–914.

Miller E et al. (2010). Incidence of 2009 pandemic influenza A H1N1 infection in England: a cross-sectional serological study. *Lancet*, 375(9720):1100–1108.

Rowe T et al. (1999). Detection of antibody to avian influenza A (H5N1) virus in human serum by using a combination of serologic assays. *Journal of Clinical Microbiology*, 37:937–943.

Ryan-Poirier KA et al. (1992). Application of Directigen Flu-A for the detection of influenza A virus in human and nonhuman specimens. *Journal of Clinical Microbiology*, 30:1072–1075.

Sanchez-Fauquier AM et al. (1991). Conservation of epitopes recognized by monoclonal antibodies against the separated subunits of influenza hemagglutinin among type A viruses of the same and different subtypes. *Archives of Virology*, 116:285–293.

Spada B (1991). Comparison of rapid immunofluorescence assay to cell culture isolation for the detection of influenza A and B viruses in nasopharyngeal secretions from infants and children. *Journal of Virological Methods*, 33:305–310.

Ukkonen P, Julkunen I (1987). Preparation of nasopharyngeal secretions for immunofluorescence by one-step centrifugation through Percoll. *Journal of Virological Methods*, 15:291–301.

Use of influenza rapid diagnostic tests
http://apps.who.int/tdr/publications/tdr-research-publications/rdt_influenza/pdf/rdt_influenza.pdf

Uyeki T (2003). Influenza diagnosis and treatment in children. A review of studies on clinically useful tests and antiviral treatment for influenza. *The Pediatric Infectious Disease Journal*, 22:164–177.

Vareckova E, Cox N, Klimov A (2002). Evaluation of the subtype specificity of monoclonal antibodies raised against H1 and H3 subtype of human influenza A virus hemagglutinins. *Journal of Clinical Microbiology*, 40:2220–2223.

Walls HH et al. (1986). Characterization and evaluation of monoclonal antibodies developed for typing influenza A and influenza B viruses. *Journal of Clinical Microbiology*, 23: 240–245.

Waner JL et al. (1990). Comparison of Directigen RSV with viral isolation and direct immunofluorescence for the identification of respiratory syncytial virus. *Journal of Clinical Microbiology*, 28:480–483.

Waner JL et al. (1991). Comparison of Directigen Flu-A with viral isolation and direct immunofluorescence for the rapid detection and identification of influenza A virus. *Journal of Clinical Microbiology*, 29:479–482.

Waris M et al. (1990). Rapid detection of respiratory syncytial virus and influenza A virus in cell cultures by immunoperoxidase staining with MAbs. *Journal of Clinical Microbiology*, 28:1159–1162.

WHO (1992). Use of monoclonal antibodies for rapid diagnosis of respiratory viruses: Memorandum from a WHO meeting. *Bulletin of the World Health Organization*, 70:699–703.

Zambon M et al. (2001). Diagnosis of influenza in the community. Relationship of clinical diagnosis of confirmed virological, serologic, or molecular detection of influenza. *Archives of Internal Medicine*, 161:2116–2122.

Ziegler T et al. (1995). Type- and subtype-specific detection of influenza viruses in clinical specimens by rapid culture assay. *Journal of Clinical Microbiology*, 33:318–321.

A(H5) outbreaks

Bender C et al. (1999). Characterization of the surface proteins of influenza A(H5N1) viruses isolated from humans in 1997–1998. *Virology*, 254:115–123.

Briand S, Fukuda K (2009). Avian Influenza A (H5N1) Virus and 2 Fundamental Questions. *Journal of Infectious Diseases*, 199(12):1717–1719.

Lin YP et al. (2000). Avian-to-human transmission of H9N2 subtype influenza A viruses: relationship between H9N2 and H5N1 human isolates. *Proceedings of the National Academy of Sciences of the United States of America*, 97:9654–9658.

Subbarao K et al. (1998). Characterization of an avian influenza A(H5N1) virus isolated from a child with a fatal respiratory illness. *Science*, 279:393–396.

Webster RG (2002). The importance of animal influenza for human disease. *Vaccine*, 20(Suppl. 2):S16–S20.

Haemagglutination and haemagglutination inhibition

Burnett FM, Stone JD (1947). The receptor destroying enzyme of Vibrio cholerae. *The Australian Journal of Experimental Biology and Medical Science*, 25:227–233.

Cox NJ, Brammer TL, Regnery HL (1994). Influenza: global surveillance for epidemic and pandemic variants. *European Journal of Epidemiology*, 10:467–470.

Cox NJ et al. (1993). Evolution of hemagglutinin in epidemic variants and selection of vaccine viruses. In: Hannoun C et al., eds. *Options for the control of influenza II*. Proceedings of the International Conference, Courchevel, Savoie, France, 27 September–02 October 1992. Amsterdam, Elsevier, 223–230.

Freshney RI (2005). *Culture of animal cells: a manual of basic technique* (5th ed.). Hoboken, NJ, Wiley-Liss.

Kendal AP, Pereira MS, Skehel J (1982). *Concepts and procedures for laboratory-based influenza surveillance*. Geneva, World Health Organization. (Copies available from the WHO Collaborating Centre for Surveillance, Epidemiology and Control of Influenza, CDC, Atlanta, GA.

Lennette, EH, Lennette, DA Lennette, ET, eds. (1995). *Diagnostic procedures for viral, rickettsial and chlamydial infections* (7th ed.). Washington, DC, American Public Health Association, 633.

Rota PA et al. (1990). Cocirculation of two distinct evolutionary lineages of influenza type B viruses since 1983. *Virology*, 175:59–68.

Shortridge KF, Lansdell A (1972). Serum inhibitors of A2-Hong Kong influenza virus haemagglutination. *Microbios*, 6:213–219.

Molecular analysis

Bustin SA, ed. (2004). A–Z of Quantative PCR (IUL Biotechnology Series). LaJolla, CA, International University Line.

CDC protocol of realtime RTPCR for influenza A (H1N1) 2009:
www.who.int/csr/resources/publications/swineflu/realtimeptpcr/en/index.html

Cheng PKC et al. (2009). Oseltamivir- and Amantadine-Resistant Influenza Viruses A (H1N1). *Emerging Infectious Diseases*, 15(6):966–968.

Daum LT et al. (2002). Genetic and antigenic analysis of the first A/New Caledonia/20/99-like H1N1 influenza isolates reported in the Americas. *Emerging Infectious Diseases*, 8(4):408–412.

Felsenstein J (1988). Phylogenies from molecular sequences: inference and reliability. *Annual Review of Genetics*, 22:521–565.

Garten RJ et al. (2009). Antigenic and genetic characteristics of swine-origin 2009 A(H1N1) influenza viruses circulating in humans. *Science*, 325:197–201.

Good laboratory practise when performing molecular amplification assays:
http://www.hpa-standardmethods.org.uk/documents/qsop/pdf/qsop38.pdf

Guo L et al. (2009). Rapid identification of oseltamivir-resistant influenza A(H1N1) viruses with H274Y mutation by RT-PCR/restriction fragment length polymorphism assay. *Antiviral Research*, 82(1):29–33.

Klimov AI et al. (1995). Prolonged shedding of amantadine-resistant influenza A viruses by immunodeficient patients: detection by polymerase chain reaction-restriction analysis. *The Journal of Infectious Diseases*, 172:1352–1355.

Mackay IM, Arden KE, Nitsche A (2002). Real-time PCR in virology. *Nucleic Acids Research*, 30(6):1291–1305.

Mullis KB (1990). The unusual origin of the polymerase chain reaction. *Scientific American*, 262(4):56–61; 64–65.

Poon LLM et al. (2009). Molecular Detection of a Novel Human Influenza (H1N1) of Pandemic Potential by Conventional and Real-Time Quantitative RT-PCR Assays. *Clinical Chemistry*, 55(8):1555–1558.

Sambrook J, Russell D (2001). *Molecular cloning: a laboratory manual* (3rd ed.). Cold Spring Harbor, NY, Cold Spring Harbor Laboratory Press, 2344.

Wang R, Taubenberger JK (2010). Methods for molecular surveillance of influenza. *Expert Review of Anti-Infective Therapy*, 8:517–527.

Weinberg GA et al. (2004). Superiority of reverse-transcription polymerase chain reaction to conventional viral culture in the diagnosis of acute respiratory tract infections in children. *The Journal of Infectious Diseases*, 189:706–710.

WHO information for laboratory diagnosis of pandemic (H1N1) 2009 virus in humans – revised:
www.who.int/csr/resources/publications/swineflu/diagnostic_recommendations/en/index.html

Wilson IA, Skehel JJ, Wiley DC (1981). Structure of the haemagglutinin membrane glycoprotein of influenza virus at 3 Å resolution. *Nature*, 289(5796):366–373.

ANNEXES

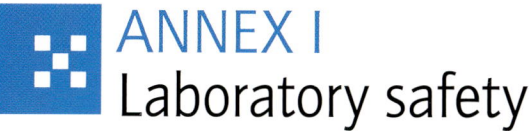
ANNEX I
Laboratory safety

Safety is the responsibility of **everybody** working in the laboratory and safe procedures must be adhered to **at all times**. Biosafety publications are included in the bibliography of the manual.

The basic rules of laboratory safety include:

- Precautions must be consistently taken when handling all clinical specimens (including blood and other bodily fluids) or other potentially infectious material (*Universal precautions*).
- Barrier protection (such as laboratory coats, gloves and other appropriate equipment) must be used at all times.
- Good general laboratory practices (such as the prohibiting of eating, drinking and smoking) should be strictly observed.
- Mechanical pipetting devices should be used for all liquids in the laboratory, as mouth pipetting is dangerous.
- Biosafety level II practices should be followed when handling all specimens.
- A class-I or class-II biosafety cabinet (or other physical containment devices) should be used for all manipulations that could produce splashes or aerosols of infectious materials.
- Adequate and conveniently located biohazard containers should always be available for the safe disposal of contaminated materials.
- Bench-tops and the surfaces of biological safety cabinets should be routinely wiped with a disinfectant (preferably 0.5% sodium hypochlorite) after each session of working with infectious agents or clinical specimens.
- **Hands should be washed frequently, especially before leaving the laboratory and before eating – protective clothing should also be removed before leaving the laboratory.**

Hazardous chemicals

- **Acetone** – used for the fixation of cell cultures in the microneutralization assay and in immunofluorescence staining.
  Caution: extremely flammable as both liquid and vapour, and harmful if inhaled.
  Eye and skin contact: flush immediately with plenty of water. Remove contaminated clothing and shoes. Seek medical attention.
  Inhalation: remove the affected person to fresh air. Seek immediate medical attention.

- **Butanol** – used as a solvent.
  Caution: extremely flammable, and harmful if inhaled, ingested or adsorbed through the skin.
  Eye and skin contact: flush immediately with plenty of water. Remove contaminated clothing and shoes. Seek medical attention.
  Inhalation: remove the affected person to fresh air. Seek immediate medical attention.
  Ingestion: seek medical advise immediately. Do not induce vomiting.

- **Ethidium bromide** – an intercalating dye used to visualize DNA in agarose gels.
  Caution: a powerful mutagen and moderately toxic. Gloves should be worn when working with solutions containing this dye, and a mask should be used when weighing it out.
  Eye and skin contact: flush with water for at least 15 minutes. Wash skin with soap and water. Seek medical attention.
  Inhalation: remove the affected person to fresh air. Give oxygen if breathing becomes difficult. Seek immediate medical attention.

- **Hydrogen peroxide** – used as a substrate for the horseradish peroxidase conjugate in immunoperoxidase staining in the ELISA phase of the neutralization test.
  Caution: may cause severe irritation of skin, eyes and mucous membranes, and respiratory irritation.
  Eye and skin contact: flush immediately with plenty of water. Seek immediate medical attention.
  Inhalation: remove the affected person to fresh air and give oxygen if breathing becomes difficult. **DO NOT ATTEMPT MOUTH-TO-MOUTH RESUSCITATION**. Seek immediate medical attention.
  Ingestion: give large volumes of water or milk if conscious. **DO NOT INDUCE VOMITING**. Seek immediate medical attention.

- **Sodium azide** – added as a preservative at a concentration of 0.1% to most of the reagents and monoclonal antibodies in the WHO Influenza Reagent Kit.
  Caution: may be fatal if swallowed, inhaled or absorbed through the skin.
  Eye and skin contact: flush with plenty of water for at least 15 minutes. Wash skin with soap and water and remove contaminated clothing. Seek immediate medical attention.
  Inhalation: remove the affected person to fresh air. Give artificial respiration or oxygen if required. Seek immediate medical attention.

ANNEX II. Cell culture inoculation and passage worksheet

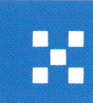

DATE: .... FLASK PASSAGE NO.: ....

Flask no.	Virus ID no.	Location/ subtype	Passage history	Vol. inoc.	Storage location	Observations							Haemagglutination test		
						Day 1	Day 2	Day 3	Day 4	Day 5	Day 6	Day 7	Turkey RBCs titre	Guinea-pig RBCs titre	Comments

Virus ID no. = virus identification number; RBCs = red blood cells; Vol. inoc. = volume inoculated.

ANNEX III. Egg inoculation record

INOCULATION								HARVEST				
DATE:								DATE:				
									Haemagglutination test titres			
Virus ID no.	Present passage	History of inoculum	Location/ subtype	Dilution	Vol. inoc.	Route of inoc.	No. of eggs inoc.	Turkey RBCs	Guinea-pig RBCs	Amn.	Allan.	Comments

Virus ID no. = virus identification number; **RBCs** = red blood cells; **Vol. inoc.** = volume inoculated; **Route of inoc.** = route of inoculation; **No. of eggs inoc.** = number of eggs inoculated; **Amn.** = amniotic fluid; Allan. = allantoic fluid.

ANNEX IV. Influenza antigen standardization worksheet

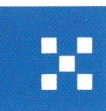

DATE: ....

No.	Antigen	Lot		Initial titre	Back titre and adjustments								
		Passage history	Date harvested		Back titration 1			Adjustment 1			Adjustment 2		
					Virus volume	PBS volume	Back titre	Virus volume	PBS volume	Back titre	Virus volume	PBS volume	Back titre

No. = number; PBS = phosphate-buffered saline.

ANNEX V
Haemagglutination inhibition test results
Field isolate identification

DATE: ....

Antigens	Laboratory identification	Reference sera					Interpretation
		1 A(H1N1) titre	2 A(H3N2) titre	3 B/Yam titre	4 B/Vic titre	5 Negative titre	
Control antigens							
A(H1N1)							
A(H3N2)							
B/Yam							
B/Vic							
Test antigens							
Field isolate 1							
Field isolate 2							
Field isolate 3							
Field isolate 4							
Field isolate 5							
Field isolate 6							
Serum control							

B/Yam = influenza B/Yamagata/16/88 lineage; B/Vic = influenza B/Victoria/02/87 lineage.

Serum identification	Date treated	Treatment method

RED BLOOD CELLS (TYPE): ....

WHO Global Influenza Programme form to accompany specimens shipped to WHOCCs

REPORTED BY: ....
Name and address of laboratory

Isolate laboratory number								
Date of specimen collection								
Patient's age								
Geographical location of patient								
Extent of influenza activity[a]								
Passage history								
Identity[b]								

[a] +++ = epidemic; ++ = localized outbreak; + = sporadic; blank = unknown.
[b] Influenza A (subtype), influenza B; blank = unknown.

Note: this form – which should accompany the specimens – should not preclude regular reporting to WHO, Geneva, Switzerland, on the Weekly Epidemiological Form No. WHO 181 for dissemination of information in the *Weekly Epidemiological Record*.

The dispatching of viruses should *not* be delayed – even if detailed epidemiological information is not yet available.

ANNEX V. HAEMAGGLUTINATION INHIBITION TEST RESULTS

ANNEXES

ANNEX VI. Haemagglutination inhibition test results
Serological diagnosis

DATE: ....

ID no.	Serum	Serum treatment	Date treated	Control antigens				Serum control	Interpretation
				A(H1N1)	A(H3N2)	B/Yam	B/Vic		
Test antisera									
1	No. 1 – S1								
2	No. 1 – S2								
3	No. 2 – S1								
4	No. 2 – S2								
5	No. 3 – S1								
6	No. 3 – S2								
7	No. 4 – S1								
8	No. 4 – S2								
Reference sera									
1	A(H1N1)								
2	A(H3N2)								
3	B/Yam/16/88 lineage								
4	B/Vic/02/87 lineage								
5	Negative control serum								

ID no. = identification number; B/Yam = influenza B/Yam/16/88 lineage; B/Vic = influenza B/Vic/02/87 lineage; S1 = acute-phase (or first) serum; S2 = convalescent-phase (or second) serum.

Control antigens	Lot no.	HA titre

Lot no. = Lot number; HA titre = haemagglutinin titre.
RED BLOOD CELLS (TYPE): ....

ANNEX VII
Microneutralization assay process sheet

Experiment name:		Experiment number:	
Investigators (List names):			
Investigators (List names):			

Part 1: Neutralization

A. Serum evaluation: Note haemolysis or lipaemia.

Use Attachment 1: Sera Condition Comments below if needed

B. Virus diluent buffer

Component	Supplier	Cat. #	Lot #	Expiration date
Dulbecco's Modified Eagle Medium (D-MEM)	Invitrogen	11965-092		
10 000 U/ml penicillin; 10 000ug/ml streptomycin	Invitrogen	15140-122		
Bovine Serum Albumin (BSA)	Roche	03117332001		
Hepes Buffer Solution (1M)	Invitrogen	15630-080		
Prepared by (Initials):		Date:		

C. Sera + Virus incubation: Record virus incubation elapsed time

Elapsed time: (1h ± 5 min)	☐ √ if 1h ± 5 min	Other: (Record)	

D. MDCK cells – Trypsin incubation

Component	Supplier	Cat. #	Lot #	Expiration date
Trypsin-EDTA	Invitrogen	25300-054		
Elapsed time: (8–10 min)	☐ √ if 8–10 min	Other: (Record)		

E. MDCK cells – count

Passage	Cell Viability	Initial Conc. of Cells		Final Vol. VD	Final Conc. ~1.5 X 10^5 cells/ml
#................................. Note: Passage # must be less than 26.	%	cells/ml		ml	
	Method used (Check):	☐ Cell Counter	☐ Haemacytometer		

F. Sera + Virus + MDCK cell incubation start time

Start time:	

G. Initials of testing operators at Day 1

Investigator	Initials:		Date:	
Investigator	Initials:		Date:	
Investigator	Initials:		Date:	

Part 2: ELISA

A. MDCK cell incubation stop time

Stop time:		Elapsed time: (18-20h)		☐ √ if 18-20h Record if other:

B. Fixation of plates incubation:

Elapsed time: (10-12 min)	☐ √ if 10-12 min	Other: (Record)	
Check cell monolayer. Record any problem wells on Attachment 2: Cell Confluence Table below if needed.			

C. 1° Antibody (Anti-NP mouse monoclonal Ab)

1° Antibody Supplier and Cat. #		1° Antibody Lot #	Working Dilution	1° Antibody Expiration date
Millipore Cat. # MAB8257 Pool Millipore Cat. # MAB8258				NA
Elapsed Time: (1h ± 5 min)	☐ √ if 1h ± 5 min	Other: (Record)		

D. 2° Antibody (Anti-mouse IgG HRP labeled) incubation:

2° Antibody Supplier and Cat. #		2° Antibody Lot #	Working Dilution	2° Antibody Expiration date
KPL Cat. # 074-1802				
Elapsed Time: (1h ± 5 min)	☐ √ if 1h ± 5 min	Other: (Record)		

E. Substrate:

Citrate Buffer (Sigma-Aldrich Cat. # P4922)	Lot#:	OPD (Sigma-Aldrich Cat. # P8287)	Lot #
	Exp. Date:		Exp. Date:

F. Initials of testing operators at Day 2:

Investigator	Initials:		Date:	
Investigator	Initials:		Date:	
Investigator	Initials:		Date:	

Part 3: Components

A. Microtitre plates

Component	Supplier	Cat. Part #	Lot #	Expiration date
Microtitre plates	Thermo Scientific	3455		

B. PBS

Phosphate Buffered Saline	Lot #	Expiration date
☐ CDC SRP Cat. # CP0549		
☐ CDC Cat. # 4550C		
☐ Other:		

Part 4: Final Review

| Reviewer Signature: | | Date: | |

Attachment 1: Sera Condition Comments

See Section 1A

CUID	Description of problem	CUID	Description of problem

Attachment 2: Cell Confluence Table

See Section 2B

List Plate #	Problem Wells	Description of problem	List Plate #	Problem Wells	Description of problem

Comments:

Initial here only if Attachment 1 or 2 is used (see Section 1A or 2B)

Investigator initials/date:	
Investigator initials/date:	

ANNEX VIII
Calculation of neuraminidase inhibition titre (NAI$_{50}$)

RECORD SHEET VIII-A
Neuraminidase activity titration

Sample	Tube number	Dilution	OD$_{549}$
Viral isolate 1	1	0	
	2	2	
	3	4	
	4	8	
	5	16	
	6	32	
	7	64	
	8	128	
Viral isolate 2	9	0	
	10	2	
	11	4	
	12	8	
	13	16	
	14	32	
	15	64	
	16	128	
Virus control	17	0	
	18	2	
	19	4	
	20	8	
	21	16	
	22	32	
	23	64	
	24	128	
Fetuin control	25	–	
	26	–	

RECORD SHEET VIII-B
Neuraminidase inhibition test results

Antigen	Working dilution	Reference antiserum	Lot no.
Viral isolate 1		Antiserum 1	
Viral isolate 2		Antiserum 2	
Viral control		Antiserum 3	

Antigen	Tube no.	Antiserum 1 Dilution	Antiserum 1 OD_{549}	Tube no.	Antiserum 2 Dilution	Antiserum 2 OD_{549}	Tube no.	Antiserum 3 Dilution	Antiserum 3 OD_{549}
Virus isolate 1	1	10		16	10		31	10	
	2	40		17	40		32	40	
	3	160		18	160		33	160	
	4	640		19	640		34	640	
	5	2560		20	2560		35	2560	
Virus isolate 2	6	10		21	10		36	10	
	7	40		22	40		37	40	
	8	160		23	160		38	160	
	9	640		24	640		39	640	
	10	2560		25	2560		40	2560	
Virus control	11	10		26	10		41	10	
	12	40		27	40		42	40	
	13	160		28	160		43	160	
	14	640		29	640		44	640	
	15	2560		30	2560		45	2560	

Antigen	OD_{549} Working dilution	½ working dilution	¼ working dilution	⅛ working dilution
Viral isolate 1				
Viral isolate 2				
Virus control				

TABLE VIII-A
Example of calculations to determine neuraminidase inhibition titres

Serum dilution ($\log_{10}$)	OD_{549} Virus + immune serum	OD_{549} Virus + negative control serum	Neuraminidase activity (%)
1.0	0.046	0.862	5
1.5	0.052	0.864	6
2.0	0.060	0.902	7
2.5	0.074	0.676	11
3.0	0.267	0.622	43
3.5	0.441	0.604	73
4.0	0.624	0.612	102

FIGURE VIII-A
Example of graph results for determining neuraminidase inhibition (NAI) titres

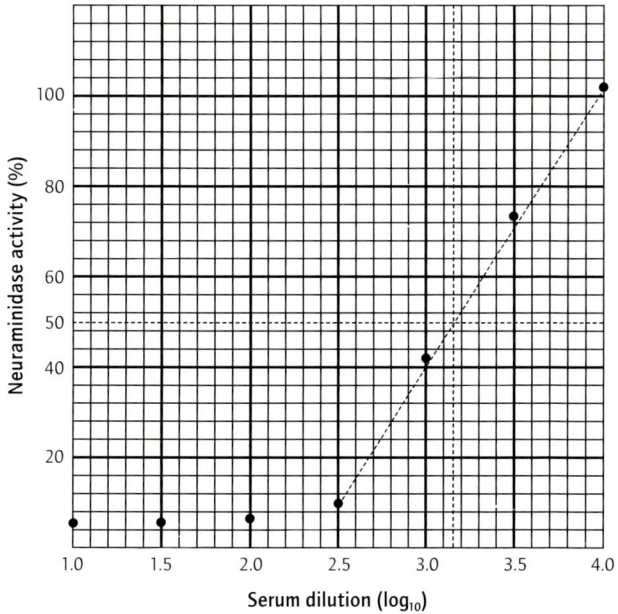

Calculations

a. Serum titre = 3.15
b. Conversion factor to 1 ml = 1.3
c. 3.15 + 1.3 = 4.45
d. Antilog_{10} 4.45 = 28 000
e. Serum NAI_{50} titre = 1:28 000